nursing
INTO THE
21st CENTURY

LEAH CURTIN

Springhouse Corporation
Springhouse, Pennsylvania

STAFF

Senior Publisher
Minnie B. Rose, RN, BSN, MEd

Clinical Consultant
Patricia Dwyer Schull, RN, MSN

Art Director
John Hubbard

Senior Associate Art Director
Stephanie Peters

Designer
Lorraine Lostracco Carbo

Associate Acquisitions Editors
Louise Quinn, Betsy K. Snyder

Editorial Assistants
Stephanie Franchetti, Jeanne Napier, A.C. Nuessle

Manufacturing
Deborah Meiris (director), Andreas Hess

For information, write Springhouse Corporation, 1111 Bethlehem Pike, P.O. Box 908, Springhouse, PA 19477-0908.

Printed in the United States of America.

NITFC-010995

℞ A member of the Reed Elsevier plc group

Library of Congress Cataloging-in-Publication Data

Curtin, Leah.
  Nursing into the 21st century / Leah Curtin.
    p. cm.
  Includes index.
    1. Nursing—United States—Forecasting.
2. Nursing—Social aspects—United States.
I. Title.
    [DNLM: 1. Nursing—trends—United States. WY 16 C978n 1996]
RT4.C87 1996
610.73—dc20
DNLM/DLC
ISBN 0-87434-834-X (alk. paper)
                                    95-595
                                    CIP

CONTENTS

32705500

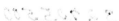

FOREWORD

Leah Curtin's pen just gets better and better.

When I am too busy to keep up with the professional literature, I steal time to read her editorials and articles. And when I vow to cut down my journal subscriptions, as I do periodically, *Nursing Management* reigns at the top of the protected list. Why? Because I know for sure I will find a gem of information on some breaking development and a point of view I need to know. And I will be amused to boot. Moreover, I never want to discard what I have read. So what could be better than a collection of Curtin's writings?

Leah is a prolific author. The selections in *Nursing into the 21st Century* cover a wide range of topics from practice and leadership to health care reform and restructuring. But Leah is no dilettante skimming the surface of a vast pond. Nor is she solely a gadfly pricking the professional conscience and then flitting off in search of another target. And, although she has the uncanny ability to point out the crux of a situation, she is more than an analyst and commentator. Leah Curtin is a seminal thinker. She is a source of new ideas. She plants new seeds in the field of ethics, which nursing and all of the health professions would do well to cultivate.

Leah may be best known to nurse managers, who have clung to her words of wit and wisdom for years. She deserves and is receiving a wider audience, because she has an important message for all who are caught up in the delivery and politics of health care. For those of us who are her followers, this compendium will serve as a ready source of refreshment. For others, it is a good introduction to a national treasure, to a fine writer, pundit, and sage.

Margretta Madden Styles

INTRODUCTION

25 YEARS OF NURSING: A SLIGHTLY IRREVERENT RETROSPECTIVE

Do you remember...a quarter of a century ago when the hospital room rate *soared* to 50 dollars a day?

• When general duty or staff nurses were rarities and team nursing was considered THE nursing care delivery system of choice?

• When most *staff* nurses were *student* nurses who were often transformed into *charge* nurses on off-shifts?

• When medical interns and residents were at least as intimidated by the nursing supervisor as staff were? (Because we suffered under the same lash, we formed alliances against the common threat — and often became life-long friends as a result of these early lessons in collaboration).

...Authority in gleaming white

Do you remember the supervisor nurse of yore? She stood five feet two inches tall and never compromised an inch. Her back was ramrod straight and her shoulders squared. Spotless white cap, gold-rimmed glasses, snow white uniform, opaque white stockings and sensible, gleaming white shoes combined to overwhelming effect.

As your pupils constricted to accommodate the glare, her features came into focus. Beneath the cap placed precisely on the crown of her head, her hair was iron gray and neatly clipped, not a hair out of place. Her jaw was square and her lips were stern. Her eyes, which twinkled bright blue behind her wire rims, conveyed intelligence and humor. Her bosom was formidable but her hips were slim: a body designed to prevent uniforms from wrinkling! Her gold nursing pin was placed neatly above the name tag over her left breast. The tag read: MISS SMITH, R.N., NURSING SUPERVISOR.

To see her was to respect her.

Supervisor Nurse (the original title of *Nursing Management*) was named for her. The journal changed, and the name changed, because the "supervisor" changed, mostly for the better. There are times, however, when I miss the "Miss Smiths" of 25 years ago. They taught me the heart and soul of nursing. We cannot bring her back—and we probably should not—but she's worth remembering.

And, by the way, do you remember...

...back to those dear, dead days *before* the hated time clock? (Who needed time clocks when you didn't pay students anyway? General duty nurses, i.e., graduates who actually **were** paid, simply worked until they were done: it never crossed anyone's mind to pay them overtime. So, of course, there was no need for a time clock.)

Do you remember when many directors of nursing withdrew from the *American Nurses Association* (ANA) because of its position on collective bargaining? They formed the *American Society of Hospital Nursing Service Administrators of the American Hospital Association.* Meanwhile, *Supervisor Nurse* added Aaron Levenstein's column on "The Art and Science of Management" to its regular features. As both lawyer and humanist, this former member of the *National Labor Relations Board* (NLRB) counseled nursing supervisors each month.

When the ANA rescinded its "no strike" clause, Dr. Levenstein wrote: "The amendment of the *Taft-Hartley Act* in 1974...will have profound effect on the nursing profession...To begin, the NLRB...has made it clear that nursing is a profession entitled to special rights in the matter of union representation...as collective bargaining spreads, hospital management will find that it can keep its legitimate prerogatives...only if it utilizes all of its

> **As the director of nursing shed her title to assume a corporate position, she also shed her uniform; a move soon followed by other nurses.**

resources in making policy...the most under-used resource is the knowledge of how work is being done in the hospital—a knowledge that is uniquely available to nursing service. [It] will force hospital administration to give greater recognition to the Director of Nursing when the chips are down."

And indeed it did. Directors of nursing soon became vice presidents of nursing. As the director of nursing shed her title to assume a corporate position, she also shed her uniform; a move soon followed by other nurses. And loud, indeed, was the lament.

The "Miss Smiths" of this world were *appalled* as younger generations of nurses slid into slacks and sneakers. Letters to the editor flew to most major journals, editors attacked the issue and researchers studied the effect of dress on professional image. As hospitals responded to the growing ranks of "flower children" among their nursing staff, dress and dress codes became matters for collective bargaining!

If "dress codes" relaxed, one can only say that communications became downright familiar. *Nursing Management's* editor commented: "While it is true that we live in an age of instant intimacy, it is also true that intimacy is reserved to one's private life. By definition, one's *professional* life is public. Thus, at the very least, public manners should prevail...I am sufficiently old-fashioned to cringe when I hear nurses introduce themselves as follows: 'Hi! I'm Nancy, I'm your nurse!' The mind boggles at the thought of a physician introducing himself in like manner: 'Hi! I'm Dickie, I'm your doc.' Or a lawyer greeting a client with 'Hi! I'm Larry the lawyer.' One need not insist on the use of a title. One could use both names: 'Hello, I am Nancy Smith. I am your nurse.'

The image of nursing

Ever since a couple of sociological studies showed that the entertainment media portrayed nurses as sex objects, nursing's "image problem" focused almost exclusively on the sex-ploitation of the profession. Nurses' indignation was almost knee-jerk predictable:

"We are *not* sex objects," we proclaimed.

The year was 1983, and it was impossible to find an October issue of *Playboy* magazine. Why? Because it featured a 10-page display on "Women in Nursing." Naturally, hardly anyone read the few words which surrounded the pictures. Feeling was running high, and nurses bought *Playboy* magazine by the carload and wrote letters to its editors by the bushel. The gist of these letters was that nurses are hard working and devoted to their jobs. They wear flat shoes and starched pinafores over their flat chests. "Visit your local hospital," we challenged them, "and you will not find one nurse who bears any resemblance whatsoever to those women in *Playboy*."

> **To say the least, if you need a meeting, you can find one today – anytime and everywhere.**

Actually, few nurses objected to being sex objects (go ahead, America, eat your heart out). They did not mind if people wanted to think nurses are beautiful and desirable and even sexy. But we did resent it when nurses were portrayed as bimbos on the boob tube: that hurt—and it undermined the credibility of the profession. Ben Casey, MD, was a sex object, but he also was the best doctor who ever lived. He was doing heart transplants in 1960— on Tuesdays. On Wednesdays he did brain surgery; on Thursdays he delivered babies in the ghetto!

We had a point—and we made one. On February 28, 1990, organized nursing launched a major campaign to enhance the image of the nurse. It succeeded—enrollments in nursing schools increased, and more opportunities than ever before opened to nurses—especially nurses in advanced practice.

Contentious fragmentation

Nursing was thrown into a tumult in the early 70s as ANA's unionization efforts—and the alliance of nursing managers with hospital

administration—deeply divided nurses. With specialty organizations proliferating, each to address a distinct area of practice, nursing leaders gave speech after speech
about the splintering profession. This,
however, did not make nurses or
nursing organizations any less frac-
tious. Finally, the *American Association
of Critical Care Nurses* called the
groups together and eventually the
*National Federation of Specialty Nurses'
Organization and the ANA* was formed. Eventually, the ANA restructured itself and formed its own federation which included the
Nursing Organization Liaison Forum (NOLF).

**Nursing became a
house divided against
itself.**

Both groups still meet regularly. To say the least, if you need a
meeting, you can find one today—anytime and everywhere. But
don't expect to have as much fun as Edith Lewis did when observ-
ing the contentious behavior of delegates at the ANA convention in
1978. Writing in *Nursing Outlook* (August 1978), Lewis commented: *It is tempting to say that the recent ANA convention was for the
birds, as they were certainly evident everywhere one walked or sat, ate
or drank. But there were birds—and birds...Particularly prominent at
this last convention was the Parliamentary Wrangler. This bird seems to
have been very busy procreating over the past two years, for it was present in greater numbers than ever before...The Red-Penciled Nitpicker
(also known as the Amendment-Amender or the Rewrite Specialist) is a
ubiquitous bird, its range of operations not limited to conventions...It is
particularly prevalent there, though, and—like the Parliamentary
Wrangler—tends to congregate with its kind around the
microphones...The Tunnel-Visioned Crusader keeps sounding a single
monotonous theme, regardless of what the other birds are chirping about;
it is a self-appointed, one-bird lobby in behalf of what it perceives to be a
neglected issue, subgroup, or special interest within the profession or,
indeed, the world...Certain birds, of course, are indigenous to the convention locale, which enabled me to spot this time, the Hawaiian Muu-*

Muu. It is an exotic bird, indeed, with brightly colored, floral-patterned plumage which seems to envelop almost its entire body...Fond of alcoholic beverages, it favors the Mai-Tai. It's a happy bird, occasionally waggling its rump in a hula-like fashion and caroling "Aloha" over and over again.

Speaking of editors

Sitting in the back of room after room, taking notes at convention after convention, the editors of several of nursing's major journals decided to take matters into their own hands.

Meeting on the sly, rebellious nursing editors formed their own "group" in 1981, carefully crafting the name to produce an appropriate acronym. Thus, the *International Academy of Nursing Editors* (INANE) formed. The first official meeting, hosted by Thelma Schorr of *The American Journal of Nursing*, consisted of two gallons of wine, munchies, and editors from nursing journals around the world swapping opinions on how to solve nursing's problems.

Today, of course, it has become quite respectable, with CEUs and formal programming. Earnest newcomers tried to reform the acronym in 1993—INANE didn't seem dignified enough. They failed, but probably not for long.

Fortunately, the proliferation of nursing organizations coincided with the move toward mandatory continuing education in nursing which started in the early 1970s and more or less ran out of steam by the mid-1980s. This is not to say that nurses are no longer required to earn CEUs. Quite the opposite. Gather ye those CEUs.

Bickering over baccalaureates

Few issues in the last 25 years have been as divisive for nursing as what came to be known as **"entry-into-practice."** When the ANA passed the "1985 RESOLUTION" calling for a minimum of a baccalaureate in nursing by the year 1985, diploma educators took up arms. When the *National League for Nursing* followed suit in 1982, the battle was engaged in earnest. And nursing became a house divided against itself.

There were, however, a few diplomats seeking, albeit unsuccessfully, to make peace. In 1979, I participated in a forum in Hartford, Connecticut, on entry into practice. One of the nurses there was 86 years old. She was still practicing nursing, although she admitted that she recently had cut back to four days a week because her knees were giving out. She worked in a nursing home and took pride in the care she gave "the poor old dears." (I suspect that she herself was older than most of her patients!) At any rate, she came to the forum to find out what "all you youngsters are in a flap about." She listened attentively to each protagonist all day. Finally, she asked if she could have her "say." As nearly as I can remember it, this is what she said:

> **Diploma schools started closing, one after another as their potential students were recruited into associate degree programs—and as funding for education was stripped out of hospital budgets by DRGs.**

When I graduated from nursing—long before most of you or even your parents were born—my class was among the first which was required to have a high school diploma before entering our two-year nurses' training program. Most of the nurses before us only had eighth-grade educations. I don't suppose we thought about it much, but I guess we were a real threat to them. Most of us were working too hard—what with the War (i.e., World War I) and everything—to worry about it. Shortly after that, sometime in the 1920s maybe, someone decided that nurses needed three years of training beyond high school—and I can't recall that too many of us disagreed. Things stayed pretty much the same for the next 20 years or so until World War II came along. We were so short of nurses in the civilian sector that we started training some women to work under nurses to help them out; we called them practical nurses because they did so many practical chores for us. It's about 35 years since then—and another 20 since nurses had to increase their training to three years. All in all that's 55 years of history. And they have been busy years: we've invented IVs and penicillin and EKGs and CT scanners and the Lord alone knows how many drugs and such. It doesn't seem to me that one extra year for RNs and for those who work under them is all that much considering that they've got to squeeze over 50 years of learning into it....

Unfortunately, however, there were far many more "agitators" both inside and outside the profession than there were peacemakers. Both the *American Medical Association* (AMA) and the *American Hospital Association* (AHA) took strong stands in favor of diploma education. Things more or less came to a head when the *New Jersey Nurses' Association* rescinded the 1985 proposal in the Fall of 1979—not by will, but by force of main strength reportedly organized and financed by the *New Jersey Hospital Association* and the *New Jersey Association of Diploma Schools*. Over 1,000 nurses hastily joined the association and were bused to the convention site for the sole purpose of forcing their professional organization to say that nurses don't need baccalaureate education. These 1,000 or so nurses were given strict written instructions as to their conduct. They were **not** to address issues and they were told **how** to vote on specific resolutions. They sat in contingents with a leader who wore white gloves and raised her gloved hand to signal the vote.

It was very exciting! Someone even stole this editor's notebook!

The fact that two-year associate degree programs had been springing up all over the country did not help matters for the diploma advocates. Diploma schools started closing, one after another as their potential students were recruited into associate degree programs—and as funding for education was stripped out of hospital budgets by DRGs.

Entry into practice is still an issue—nurses rarely let go of anything—but other matters took center stage as the drive to control health costs began to dominate the political scene.

Physicians and nurses: shoulder to shoulder...and head to head

From the time of Nightingale onward, nurses and physicians had their differences. The Physicians of Her Majesty's Army *did not* want Nightingale in the Crimea and tried for all they were worth to keep her out. When that did not work, they tried to force her out. Unreasonable restrictions, refusal of access to the wounded, diseased quarters (in fact, the whole "hospital" was built over an open sewer) were all calculated to discourage Nightingale and her small cadre of nurses. It was the common soldiers whose lives were saved or whose dying they made easier who supported them. It was the war correspondents who wrote of their heroism, who rallied public support for the nurses. Of course, it was Ms. Nightingale's steely will which finally won the day. By the time Nightingale left the Crimea, the Surgeon General himself *did not issue an order unless it was countersigned by her.*

With this glorious start, nurses marched confidently into the 20th century, changing and reforming every system they touched. Thus, in the early 1970s, when the *American Medical Association* suggested that 100,000 nurses be *upgraded* to physician assistants, the *American Nurses Association* responded that nurses already did assist physicians and they certainly did not need to be upgraded to do so. The AMA countered by creating physician assistants (PAs) and the ANA, in its turn, created the nurse practitioner (NP). And the battle was joined once again.

Physician and nurse peacemakers soon founded the *National Joint Practice Commission* (NJPC) which was supported by grants and funding from both associations. The various site projects were quite successful, but the NJPC went defunct when AMA withdrew its support in the early 80s. Not surprisingly, nurses went on to promote "independent" practice and third-party reimbursement for their services while the AMA fumed and fought them every inch of the way.

By the mid to late 80s, a nursing shortage loomed on the horizon—and the AMA responded with what came to be known as the *RCT PROPOSAL*. The AMA proposed that physicians train high school graduates to give patient care, that these trainees take tests and be registered in their states, and that the registered care technologist report directly to the physician. The ANA, in fact all nurses, practically gobbled in outrage. Few things have so united the nursing profession. In one strong voice, nurses said NO.

In 1990, with health reform looming on the horizon, nurses proposed—and have garnered great support from politicians and the general public—that nurse practitioners provide the bulk of primary care in America. They would work in partnership with primary care physicians, but they would not be subordinate to them. Physicians and nurses would go *head to head* on this one, but the nurses will probably "win" because they really **are** competent—and the physicians who work with them know it and value it.

The cornerstone of the government's new prospective payment plan was the Diagnostic Related Groups (DRGs) concept originally developed at Yale University as a management and utilization review tool.

However, physicians are gun-shy: they watched nurse anesthetists initiate their role and improve their credentials. It wasn't until the late 1980s, when nurse anesthetists fought for and won third-party reimbursement, that anesthesiologists woke up to the fact that nurse anesthetists provided the bulk of anesthesia services in the United States.

Nurse midwives, long maligned by the medical profession, also are coming into prominence, particularly as a malpractice crisis drove many physicians out of obstetrics. The rapid growth of uninsured pregnant women combined with this shortage of obstetricians to telling effect: many obstetricians are seeking nurse midwives to work with them in their practice, or providing backup for them in obstetrical clinics located in underserved areas.

> **Assets and functions were transferred to produce better results, and new functions (both provider and non-provider) were spun off as soon as financially, legally and operationally possible.**

Despite the thunder and lightning at the national level flashing and crashing between physician's *organizations* and nurse's *organizations*, nurses and physicians at the point of care work well together. In fact, most nurse practitioners work in physicians' offices. Almost all physicians who have worked with them strongly support professional nurse case managers. Moreover, when it comes to the quality of a patient's care, nurses and physicians almost always stand shoulder to shoulder.

Ushering in an era of competition

On December 28, 1982, Mr. Secretary Schweiker, in his "Report to Congress on Hospital Prospective Payment for Medicare," shed considerable light on the impact and provisions of the *Tax Equity and Fiscal Responsibility Act of 1982*, also known as TEFRA.

The cornerstone of the government's new prospective payment plan was the Diagnostic Related Groups (DRGs) concept originally developed at Yale University as a management and utilization review tool. To put it simply, the patient population was divided into Major Diagnostic Categories (MDCs), which were further subdivided into 356 DRGs, subdivided again according to age and the presence or absence of complications. A dollar figure, based on retrospective cost data for a hospital and region, was derived by averaging the cost of the care given to patients who have had this diagnosis, adjusted to account for inflation plus one percent. (This latter provision was routinely reversed in following years.) A hospital's income for Medicare is determined by dividing the allowable Medicare costs assigned to each DRG by the number of patients discharged who have been assigned to that DRG.

Unfortunately, when whatever it is that hits the fan actually hits it, the results rarely are evenly distributed. Some 100 hospitals closed their doors as a result of DRGs, but by 1993 most of the remaining hospitals were realizing unprecedented "margins". Larger teaching hospitals that give care to people who tend to have expensive things wrong with them were not hit as hard as rural community hospitals. Hospitals whose patient mix was liberally laced with people who carry private insurance simply shifted their costs. Hospitals that had elaborate computer systems in place adjusted more quickly and easily to the new federal regulations because they had easier access to the huge amount of data they need to satisfy the feds.

The implications of these and other regulatory changes—and the impact they had on nursing—were vast and varied. Without doubt, nursing managers were under heavy pressure to reduce the cost of delivering nursing care to patients. Salaries, fringe benefits, staffing ratios, absenteeism, and inefficiency were scrutinized closer than ever before. Quality assurance—the incidence of nosocomial infections, accidents and errors—assumed even more importance as the healthcare industry moved into continuous quality improvement, benchmarking, and the measurement of patients' actual outcomes.

According to L. Edward Bryant, an attorney who spoke at the 1982 *American Society of Nursing Service Administrators'* annual meeting, hospitals were to be reorganized and, in many instances, placed under the auspices of a broadly based charitable parent organization. *He was right.* Coequal with the hospital was a non-provider holding company which included a separate development foundation to raise, hold, and invest money for the hospital and other charitable services; a human services organization to provide physical therapy, rehabilitation services, education, research, community affairs, day care and so forth; and a taxable corporation which offered certain outpatient services (in competition with drugstores and appliance rental agencies), home health services (in competition with private agencies), freestanding emergicenters and surgicenters, and so forth. *He was right again.*

Assets and functions were transferred to produce better results, and new functions (both provider and non-provider) were spun off as soon as financially, legally and operationally possible. Some were dismal failures, others were successful beyond anyone's expectations.

These regulatory changes had enormous impact on the role of nurses in management and administrative positions. Up to the 1980s, most nursing managers had spent almost half their time delivering clinical care. Few had the time anymore. Instead, they planned, implemented and evaluated change; guided the professional development of staff; selected and allocated the material resources necessary for patient care; designed and implemented staffing patterns based on patient acuity; developed, presented and justified unit or area budgets; coordinated interdepartmental communications and activities; interviewed and selected personnel for their units; and participated in numerous decision-making bodies (e.g., utilization review, product review and infection control). Nurse managers also became more deeply involved in performance evaluation, policy formation, the maintenance of standards of practice, and eventually the measurement of outcomes.

Nursing executives designed new systems to control costs and assure consistency and continuity of care both inside and outside the hospital. Critical pathways which integrated nursing and medical regimens improved productivity and quality inside the hospital. Professional nurse case managers moved out into the community to coordinate the care of complicated patients, and nurse-run clinics began to appear to provide primary care.

During this period, the *American Society of Nursing Service Administrators* became the *American Organization of Nurse Executives* (AONE). At its annual meeting in 1994, the AONE membership voted to include all nurses in management positions as members. This move recognized the changes the 1980s had wrought in the nurse manager's role.

Lest we forget

There was a time well within recent memory when almost no one, not even physicians, carried malpractice insurance. Quality assurance and risk management were in their infancy. In fact, few hospitals even **had** incident report forms, and ethical "problems" were few and far between—or more precisely either unrecognized or slid under the rug.

At any rate, with increasing technology, sicker patients now survived or, in some cases, merely survived a bit longer. Their fragile, highly volatile conditions required special attention—close monitoring and a concentration of technology. Thus, critical care units were born in the 60s and "specialized" in the 70s and 80s. Because these special units gathered critically ill patients into one area, the ethical problems they presented became increasingly harder to ignore. One of the first ethical problems we could no longer ignore was the appropriate use of cardiopulmonary resuscitation (CPR).

Cardiopulmonary resuscitation was developed *primarily* to assist heart patients and those whose hearts were temporarily affected by trauma or disease. As such, it was a *life-saving* procedure. Unfortunately, many people fell victim to the notion that it could bring people **back** to life. CPR was developed to buy enough time for either surgical intervention or natural healing to occur. Nothing more. Therefore, when surgical intervention was not possible and when natural healing could not occur, the use of CPR became both inappropriate and unreasonable. However, fears of malpractice suits kept many physicians and hospitals from developing anything other than "blanket policies".

Nurses were placed in paradoxical positions by conflicting written and verbal instructions from physicians; by orders that conflicted with hospital policy; by conflicting and inter-conflicting directions from patients, family members, and physicians; by their own conflicting perceptions and values; and finally by the absence of a clear, rational, and humane hospital policy regarding CPR.

People were not allowed to *die* in hospitals; they could only experience *regulated deaths*. That is to say, individuals (or their Creator) were not permitted to disrupt hospital routine and bypass established procedures by dying on their own. The procedures, policies, and routines demanded that they be thumped, pumped, infused, wired, intubated and preferably moved to a critical care unit before death could occur. In short, people didn't die simply— they had to be processed to die.

Eventually the federal government, never loathe to step into a vacuum, passed legislation to *force* hospitals to rethink their CPR policies. *The Patient Self-Determination Act* took effect on December 1, 1991. It requires hospitals, nursing homes, and hospices to advise patients, *on admission*, of their right to accept or refuse medical treatment. Compliance with the Act became a condition of Medicare and Medicaid reimbursement.

While this helped handle some issues, ethical problems stretched far beyond CPR. Some of the most poignant dealt with infants and children.

Irreversibly dying infants

Technological advances in neonatology enabled us to save *and to cure* infants who formerly were irretrievably dying—or doomed to a life of irremedial suffering. Morbidity and mortality statistics did turn around. Tragedy often was turned into triumph. Nonetheless, there still was tragedy. The greatest tragedies *were not* those infants who must die, nor did these children present any ethical problems not faced in the past. Common sense dictates that we provide what comfort measures we can to child and parents: warmth, compassion, the touch of a hand, a little food and water if the child can eat—*nothing more nor less.*

Sadly, common sense seems to have been in woefully short supply in recent decades. Scientific and technologic imperatives—the need to learn, to experiment, to use technologically improved tools simply because they were there—far too often rode roughshod over common sense.

Far more difficult are the problems presented when advanced technology "half-way" works: when a respirator might keep a child alive, but he'll never walk free from it; when a surgical procedure may enable a child to be fed, but he'll never be conscious enough to know hunger; when infection can be treated only so that a child may live in coma; in short, when technology can be used to preserve biological life in the absence of human

> **Because these special units gathered critically ill patients into one area, the ethical problems they presented became increasingly harder to ignore.**

potential. If this could be known in advance—*and sometimes it could*—common sense precluded the use of technology to achieve so mean an end. If it could be known in advance—*and often it could*—that technological or surgical intervention yield a high probability that this will be the result, common sense leaves such decisions in the hands of parents. However, confusion about what is and is not a parental prerogative muddied the ethical waters. Many believed that the parents' decision included veto power over only the technology or the surgery; that no human being, not parent or any other, has the authority to order abandonment or death. Others disagreed.

The problem was exacerbated by the fact that none of us were too sure where common law stood on all this. To date, the courts have been clear on only one point: each case will be judged on its own merits.

In reviewing court decisions about treatment of defective newborns, it seems that they struggled to make distinctions among: 1) appropriate treatment of irreversibly dying infants; 2) appropriate treatment of infants at high risk of living a life totally devoid of meaning; and 3) appropriate treatment of infants who could live but whose lives would not be "normal." In the first two circumstances, the general thrust seemed to allocate treatment decisions to parents.

The third circumstance presented altogether different propositions. Neither the courts nor the federal government seemed inclined to treat them as purely personal matters protected by the right to privacy. These, indeed, are the classic "Baby Doe" cases. The potential for survival is high; the potential for a "normal" life is low. If the infant is treated, the parents (unless they surrender custody to the state) must carry all the responsibilities associated with rearing a handicapped child. If the child is not treated, he will die. To put the matter succinctly, the situation pits the hard-won civil rights of handicapped citizens against the traditional common law rights of parents to make decisions for their children.

> **While most of the ethical questions of the past dealt with abundance—too much treatment, a right to refuse treatment, how much is enough treatment—the problems emerging today deal with scarcity.**

Nurses, though often excluded from decision-making, were as bemused and as traumatized as the rest of the community by these tragedies. The difference was that nurses worked with the infants and often lived with the decisions of others. If the "Baby Doe" cases accomplished nothing else, they compelled health providers to establish functioning multidisciplinary ethics committees. Ethics committees, and eventually the JCAHO nursing standard which required hospitals to provide a mechanism through which nurses can mediate their ethical problems, are not perfect solutions but they are preferable to legislation.

Dr. Jack Kevorkian's recent forays into physician-assisted suicide are likely to force a *legislative* as well as a voluntary response to the ethical question of euthanasia.

Health reform 1990s style

While most of the ethical questions of the past dealt with abundance—too much treatment, a right to refuse treatment, how much is enough treatment—the problems emerging today deal with scarcity. Debates about rationing flared as the state of Oregon sought to limit publicly financed access to high tech medical interventions **when** this was necessary to enable access to a basic package of care for all its citizens.

This debate moved to the national level in 1992 as President Clinton proposed health reform—and with it, the development of a basic package of care that would be available to all Americans. By definition, that means some treatments will be included—and some will be excluded.

People everywhere are talking about health reform: the well-insured because they fear restrictions, the uninsured because they fear exclusion. Everyone in healthcare is nervous about different things. Physicians because they are afraid their incomes will be cut and their practices controlled. Administrators because they fear reduced revenues and more regulations. Suppliers because they fear price caps or even cuts. Nurse administrators because they fear budget cuts and reduced staffing.

During any period of waiting, anxiety—fueled by fear—rises. Sometimes this leads to frenzied activity and sometimes to paralysis. Both can be fatal.

Colleagues, fear not, neither let your hearts be weary. Rejoice, I bring you glad tidings. We have spent the whole of our professional careers in a climate at least as chaotic as that created by Bill Clinton and his band of merry reformers; and I assure you, *this* not only can be endured, it can be enjoyed.

You do have to ignore a lot of stuff in order to laugh about health reform—things like being "restructured" out of your job and such—but we can conquer these worries by taking it a day at a time.

Here are three perfectly good reasons to keep laughing during health reform:

1. **Things are not getting worse.** Things have always been this bad. Few things are as consoling as the long perspective of history. It will perk you up no end to go back and read the works of retired leaders of the healthcare industry. You will learn that things back then were terrible too, and what's more, they were always getting worse. This is most inspiring.

-**Dateline: 1968.** The nation is undergoing health reform. Medicare and Medicaid begin implementation. The AMA predicts that government interference will lead to socialism. These changes turned the world of hospitals and healthcare upside down.

-**Dateline: 1982.** The nation is undergoing health reform again. Congress passed DRG legislation. Hospitals become competitive organizations. Physicians et al. become entrepreneurs. The AMA claims that the whole system is going to hell in a handbasket and we'll be socialized before we know it. These changes turned the world of hospitals and healthcare upside down.

-**Dateline: 1994.** The nation is undergoing health reform yet again. The Clinton Administration is pushing for "managed competition" and "global budgets" to control health costs. The AMA draws a "line in the sand" over global budgets, seeks federal antitrust relief to let physicians negotiate rates with groups, and wants change in ERISA (the Employee Retirement Income Security Act) so that self-insured benefit plans would have to negotiate with physicians. Otherwise, the AMA warns, health care will be rationed and the system inevitably will slide into socialism. These changes will turn the world of hospitals and health care upside down.

2. **Things could be worse.** The fact that they probably will get worse is no excuse for tossing away this golden opportunity to rejoice in the relative delightfulness of our current situation. Is there anything to cheer us in the realization that competition in healthcare is now to be "managed" which, in turn, somehow will lead to universal access? Yes. Writing in the *Futurist* magazine (26:2), Weiner predicted that the "burgeoning health insurance crisis" will lead to "health wars" in which activists for one disease (such as breast cancer) will challenge the emphasis put on another (such as AIDS). Let us give thanks for the time "managed competition" may buy us—while we still have time.

> **Few things are as consoling as the long perspective of history. It will perk you up no end to go back and read the works of retired leaders of the healthcare industry. You will learn that things back then were terrible too, and what's more, they were always getting worse. This is most inspiring.**

3. There is always the off-chance that **adversity will improve our character.** Since we are all the spiritual children of the Puritans (though mostly "fallen-away"), we secretly believe that suffering is good for the soul. Constant chaos sort of keeps you on your toes spiritually.

From the time Clinton selected Donna Shalala to head HHS, and former CBO director Alice Rivlin coupled with Leon Panetta, House Budge Committee Chairman, to head the Office of Management and Budget, the nay-sayers have been swallowing their tongues. Managed care, global budgets, DRGs, health insurance reform, managed competition. This is great stuff even if we **do** feel as if our backs are up against the wall.

Back up against the wall

Whenever I think of someone whose "back is against the wall," I think of some of our predecessors, those early nurses who were moral, clinical and social activists. Perhaps today's nurses do not know how much they spring from these gallant women.

> **Nursing was born of one woman's dream, which became a great cause, which eventually produced a fine tradition of humanitarian service and, whatever problems we face, we are part of that living tradition.**

Modern nursing started when Nightingale began to yearn for social justice in an era of social change. She sought to improve the life of the common man and to "open a career highly paid" for the uncommon woman. She did both. In Victorian England against overwhelming odds. She and a small band of nurses whom she trained went to war. And they turned around mortality and morbidity statistics at Scutari—and, within a few decades, trained nurses turned them around in the entire Western World.

Although their backs often were against the wall, those mighty few saved and changed the lives of millions. And they went on to create a new profession, to refashion every aspect of the care of the sick, to change rules and regulations and laws. And to create new disciplines along the way. Who are the valiant women whom contemporary critics rudely (and inaccurately) dismiss as servile handmaidens?

- Florence Nightingale founded the discipline of biostatistics.
- Lillian Wald founded the first "Settlement House" for the indigent.
- Elizabeth Kinney founded the discipline of physical medicine.
- Nurses were the first women to be declared "officers and gentlemen" by an act of Congress. The first woman to hold a permanent commission in the United States Army was Colonel

Florence A. Blanchfield, Chief of the Army Nurse Corps. On June 19, 1947, she was given the United States Army serial number N-1. A total of 492 Army Nurse Corps officers were integrated into the regular army as a result of the passage of public law 36 passed on April 16, 1947.

- The statue of a nurse (Ruth Parsons) was placed in Arlington Cemetery to honor all nurses who served in the armed services, particularly those who served during times of war and who were wounded or killed.

- The nurse's chapel at Westminster Abbey was established after World War II to honor nurses killed during that conflict. It is graced by a huge stained glass window of a nurse.

- The first woman to be awarded the French Cross for bravery was the heroine of Dien Bien Phu, Genevieve de Galard-Terrause, who refused to abandon her patients (wounded French soldiers) in the face of probable death at the hands of the Viet Cong.

- Dorothea Lynde Dix, the superintendent of women nurses during the Civil War, led the drive to reform the treatment of patients in mental institutions. Educated as a teacher, Ms. Dix devoted most of her later life to nursing the ill, protecting their rights and humanizing their treatment.

- Margaret Sanger, RN, a public health nurse in New York City, started the woman's health movement.

Moreover, I haven't even scratched the surface of nurses' accomplishments. And our profession is only about 140 years old, a mere infant as professions go. Our predecessors were vigorous, positive, effective achievers. Nursing was born of one woman's dream, which became a great cause, which eventually produced a fine tradition of humanitarian service and, whatever problems we face, we are part of that living tradition.

There are worse places to be than with our backs against the wall. In fact, that's when we do our best.

From command to negotiation

Our traditions led to yet more changes in nursing's management role. Health networks—clinics, subacute care units, home care, hospices—now challenge managers anew to try and test different ways to integrate and deliver care.

Effective participation in multidisciplinary teams requires knowledge and appreciation of the contributions and problems of **other** professionals, technicians and departments that comprise the modern health-care network. The term "negotiation" takes on new meaning—it no longer refers only to labor-management relationships; rather, it encompasses a whole range of daily transactions.

To mediate the demands of institutional policy and clinical practice requires a high degree of sophistication—both an in-depth knowledge of what is needed for safe patient care and an in-depth knowledge of the art and science of management. To facilitate the practice of their co-workers, nurse managers must re-form and reapply administrative goals to make them relevant and achievable in each particular department. Today's complex healthcare networks require nursing managers who can motivate, assign, service, coordinate, troubleshoot and "pick up the pieces" for the highly specialized, many-ranked men and women who must work together to provide high quality **patient** care.

This is a time of transition for both professions and institutions: conflicting tensions and interprofessional stress demand that nursing's leaders at all organizational levels exhibit patience, knowledge, skill, tact, humor and grace under pressure. Nursing's management role has grown and changed, and nurse managers often must function as self-contained, on-the-spot decision processors and action facilitators.

From the editor's desk

"Who hasn't been moaning about the pace of change?" *Supervisor Nurse's* founding editor, Dorothy Kelly, wrote after reading Alvin

Toffler's newly published book, *Future Shock*. She suggested that each of us build "stability zones" as permanent or temporary relief from too many and too rapid changes. And that was in 1970!

In that first year, Kelly wrote: "Nursing is beginning to look like a chicken with its head cut off." And today chief nursing officers are seeing their jobs eliminated as entire nursing departments are integrated into self-directed teams. However prophetic Ms. Kelly may have been, let's hope she was wrong when she went on to say, "you don't have to come from a farm to know that the chicken eventually flops down dead."

> **"It probably doesn't matter how we do things, just so long as we keep our eye and our heart on the patients. They are the ones who need us."**

Nonetheless, a year later when Miss Lillian Wald was inducted into **The Hall of Fame for Great Americans**, Ms. Kelly opined, "Perhaps Lillian Wald operated in a simpler day. Perhaps what nursing accomplishes today must be 'the work of a committee.' It probably doesn't matter how we do things, just so long as we keep our eye and our heart on the patients. They are the ones who need us."

With these few words, she defined nursing's "stability zone." One that she—and we—held safe as the pace of change accelerated ever faster every year.

June 1994

Chapter 1

NURSES
AND
NURSING

NURSING: WHY STAY?

Anne Morrow Lindberg, in her beautiful and sensitive book, *Gift from the Sea*, wrote: "When one is a stranger to oneself, then one is estranged from others, too. If one is out of touch with oneself, then one cannot touch others...."

This thought crosses my mind again and again as I think about such television "specials" on nursing as "The Oprah Winfrey Show," *et al.* I hear and watch nurses, my colleagues, harangue and condemn, express cold resentment for patients and their needs, angrily demand *both* public pity *and* public support. I don't doubt their sincerity or even the horror stories they tell, but I think "good grief!" They've equated their worst day with their entire careers, and laid it all on the profession as a whole. Or, even more sadly, they've allowed the difficulties they've faced—and usually over-come—to rob them of a sense of their own victories: their success-es in the teeth of opposition. Resentment has eroded their own self-esteem—and their own power. And then I think, "perhaps I am out of synch—out of touch. Perhaps I have become a stranger to my own profession. Can I no longer touch my colleagues?"

Obscuring success

Is it possible that our preoccupation with the problems, obstacles and frustrations of practice has blotted out our achievements, advances and successes? Just as we all live in a physical environ-ment and adjust to its constraints, so too we live in a psychological environment that shapes the way we think. If we were living in an era of optimism, we should be more likely to see the world in rosier hues. This is an important point to remember, particularly in a period like the present when the process of selective perception filters out the positive and focuses on the negative, even seamy, side of just about everything. Recent forays into the literature of and about the nursing shortage illustrate this point. Rarely does any nurse or healthcare leader mention anything positive about the profession, or the environment, or even the patients. If you can't find something to criticize, why say anything at all?

Certainly, serious thinkers always critique prevailing practices. However, we may have gone a bit too far: we've sacrificed a balanced perspective to a desire for reform. And nurses are the casualties: robbed of their success, denied their own heritage, their self-esteem and professional pride have been shattered. And with it, our sense of power and ability to shape our own destinies. How can it be that those who "care" have been disheartened?

An ancient tradition

We in nursing share a common cause and a common tradition. It goes way back in human history to a moment when some primitive ancestor was moved to compassion by someone else's suffering. Its roots are found in this Stone Age relative's need to teach others what he or she learned from experience, trial and error, experimentation. There was no one around selling stone tablets on the subject. There wasn't even an alphabet. There was nothing but the need to help and to be helped—a need which overcame suspicion, prejudice, and even fear of plague. A need which whetted and justified a thirst for learning, knowing and understanding—and then sharing this knowledge with and for others. Our traditions, our ancestors go back to those who debrutalized Brute Man with such revolutionary intuitions as "gentleness is preferable to violence," "knowledge conquers more surely than weaponry," and "human sympathy is more important than anyone's ideology." These ancestors even noticed that brutes cannot shed tears—and it's tears that make you human.

Centuries later this knowledge and these intuitions became words intended to instruct and dignify human beings through service to—rather than ostracism of—the sick. Nursing's traditions are humanitarian in the fully philanthropic meaning of that term: love of mankind. How this "love" is best carried out for the good and welfare of the individual and of society is and has been the focus of both the philosophical thinkers and doers of our profession...so much so that we have progressed from Maimonides' (1207 AD) lowest level of charity (i.e., to give aid proportionately to the distress of those who suffer) to his highest level (i.e., to anticipate charity by preventing suffering, by teaching our neighbors to care for themselves, by rendering them independent).

A tradition with a future

We in nursing have a tradition with a future. The tender loving care of human beings (yes, I choose to use this phrase though it has become trite, even passe, in some circles) will never become obsolete. In today's strained world among tomorrow's strange machines, people *more than ever* need to be touched to be restored, renewed, revived and redeemed. Today, technology has brought us closer than ever before to the pain of living, so finally we have learned that health really does lie in restoring independence, not merely ministering to illness.

If we really believe this, then we know, as surely as anyone can know, that nurses' hands—helping hands—can also be used to help themselves. Our traditions require us to use our hands and our minds and our hearts to help others—and just as surely, they require us to help ourselves. Who—if not we—will help the helpers? heal the healers? care for the caregivers? We are a maturing profession, and part of that "growing up" is to assume the responsibility to help and heal and redeem and render ourselves independent. The nurses who cry on television are much like the adolescents who trade on, while raging about, their dependence. Independence is never a present: it's earned and it's paid for. So is pride, and achievement and success.

Why be a nurse? Why stay? You can earn a good living (nurses, on average, earn more than most female college graduates), but you could earn as much or more elsewhere. Nurses have a lot of mobility and flexibility (go anyplace—and if you're competent, you'll be welcomed with open arms), but a few other occupations offer almost as much mobility as we have. Nursing also offers a lot of variety—from school nurse to nurse anesthetist, from public health care nurse to dean of a school, from nurse midwife to career officer in the military, from flight nurse to independent practitioner, from critical care specialist to family counselor. But then, I suppose that somewhere else you'll find almost as much variety.

A tradition of success

Why stay in nursing? Why be a nurse? Well, I can only answer for myself, and even then in someone else's words. For at least two decades, for far too long, nurses have presented themselves to the public as failures—as second class—or almost, but not quite, good enough. It's a lie. Actually, nursing is one of the few things one can do to earn a living that really does offer hope for a successful life. Ralph Waldo Emerson described a genuinely successful life: "To laugh often and love much; to win the respect of intelligent persons and the affection of children; to earn the approbation of honest critics and endure the betrayal of false friends; to appreciate beauty; to find the best in others; to give of one's self, to leave the world a bit better...; to have played and laughed with enthusiasm and sung with exultation; to know even one life has breathed easier because you have lived—this is to have succeeded."

Throughout my years in nursing, this profession has provided it all:

—to love much those whose courage and strength inspire admiration.

—to laugh with them in the face of pain and even death.

—to win the respect of intelligent people who know what it takes to act with grace under pressure.

—to endure the betrayal of false friends who publicly denigrate your work.

—to find the best in others as we seek to build on their strength.

—to give of one's self even when your reserves seem depleted (Maslow's triangle really should have been a volcano, for it is only in reaching out of self that the self can be fully actualized).

—to leave the world a bit better because someone's pain was diminished, someone's sorrow comforted, someone's choice restored, someone's child did not die alone.

—to have lived with enthusiasm (how can one value life if one has never witnessed the suffering that nature can extract from one human body?)

—to know, really know, literally know that one life has breathed easier because you have lived—and known what to do, and shared and given.

If one persists in nursing with unrelenting professionalism and tenacity, success—a successful life—is assured. These are my reasons for being a nurse, for staying in nursing. They may not be the same as yours, but then, when all is said and done, maybe, just maybe, they're yours, too.

July 1988

DESIGNING NEW ROLES: NURSING IN THE 90S AND BEYOND

A wise man once said, "In today already walks tomorrow." The problem is to distinguish between what truly walks with us day after day (a trend) and what merely waltzes through for an hour or so (a fad). How can we tell the difference? Fads have no socio-economic or political roots. Trends do. To spot trends we must separate illusion from reality as dispassionately as possible. To do so successfully we must be honest.

Here's how some of the trends shaping in the '90s are shaping up for nursing and healthcare:

1. The economic boom of the 1980s was not a real boom at all. It was an illusion built on borrowing. We have a $3 trillion national debt and another $3 trillion in consumer debt. To counter this disastrous trend, economists, financiers and politicians warn that we must reduce the national debt, encourage consumer savings, increase productivity and keep taxes low to avoid a terrible depression.

What does this mean for healthcare?
- continuing pressure to lower costs.
- growth in managed care.
- rationing of access to high technology.
- increasing demands for service from the uninsured.
- an accelerating move to outpatient services.

2. The aging of the population, combined with the birth dearth of the '70s and '80s, will skew more than our demographics: marketing, politics and work values will also be skewed.

What does this mean for healthcare?
- increasing demand for convenience of time, location and service delivery.
- a shift upward in the age of patients—80 percent of the hospital census will be comprised of those over 65.

- an increasing shortage of nurses and other health workers (except MDs).
- government's share of costs will increase from about 45 percent today to over 60 percent in the next few years.
- a shift toward lower tech, higher touch, less invasive diagnostic and therapeutic interventions.

3. Environmental concerns will dominate in the '90s and focus attention on personal physical fitness, industrial health, and pollution control.

What does this mean for healthcare?

- diet and nutrition (diet is implicated in 5 of the 10 top killer diseases) will be *the* consumer focus of the '90s.
- people will seek a "back to basics" style of healthcare (not anti-tech or anti-drugs) which focuses on consumer involvement not only in decision making but also in care and treatment. Both hospitals and eldercare facilities should design their buildings and their policies with this in mind. Wholistic Care Units, combining conventional medicine with alternative care techniques (acupressure/acupuncture, biofeedback, relaxation therapy, etc.), will become popular in the latter half of the 90s.
- hospitals and healthcare providers will seek bonding relationships with business and industry—both with those for whom they provide service and with those which provide services to them. For example, managed care contracts with corporations may include commitments (a) to provide industrial health consultation, assess environmental hazards and to provide services; (b) to offer *pre-employment* history and physical exams, not only for employees but also for their families; and (c) to provide healthcare experts to teach employees/families about prevention. Companies which serve the healthcare industry (a) will be expected to provide deep discounts in exchange for long term contracts; (b) will be more deeply involved in developing and testing products in the hospital and designing inservice education programs to avoid productivity lags with the introduction of new technologies; and (c) will be expected to help bear some of the costs of indigent care.

What does all this mean for nurses?

A recent press release from the World Health Organization's Regional Office for Europe summarizes matters nicely. "There [is] a fundamental need for a clearly identifiable, skillful and dedicated health professional: the generalist nurse whose work involves the main themes of the "Health for All" movement. This person should live in the community and maintain regular contact with individuals, families and groups in their homes, schools and other institutions, workplaces and at leisure facilities... [Leaders must consider] how nursing could be strengthened to bring "health for all" into every area of peoples' life and work, and provide expertise in a broad range of health and care functions..."

For those unfamiliar with the "Health for All" movement, some of its 38 principal targets follow:

• "The first 12 targets describe the fundamental requirements for people to be healthy, which the work of nurses and midwives can help to achieve. Their completion data is the year 2000. First, *equity in health* must be ensured by reducing the differences in health status between the sexes, social and economic groups and countries. The other necessity is to strengthen health; this can be done in three ways."

"First, Targets 2 and 3 aim to *add life to years* by ensuring the full development and use of each person's physical and mental capacities to benefit from and cope with life in healthy ways. Chances for the elderly, the disadvantaged and the physically and mentally disabled to lead socially and economically fulfilling lives are particularly important."

"Targets 4 and 5 are to *add health to life* by reducing disease and disability and by eliminating some diseases (indigenous measles, poliomyelitis, neonatal tetanus, congenital rubella, diphtheria, congenital syphilis and indigenous malaria)."

"The last seven targets in this group require action to *add years to life*. Life expectancy at birth should be raised to 75 years. The rate of infant mortality in the Region should be less than 20 deaths per 1,000 live births and maternal mortality should be less than 15 per 100,000 live births. Numbers of deaths from circulatory disease, cancer and accidents, the three main killers in the Region, should be reduced, and the current increase in suicide and suicide attempts should be reversed."

- "The environment powerfully affects health, and the next group of targets concerns protecting people from health risks in the environment and improving the places where people live and work, not only to safeguard people from risks but also to promote their health by improving the quality of life."

> **The adult med-surg nurse will receive more and more attention as the vast majority of inpatient beds will be adult med-surg.**

- "Community resources in sectors other than health should be organized to work for Health for All. Because health is everybody's business, well-integrated, community-based programs that combine all aspects of primary healthcare should be set up in every community."

- "The final part of appropriate care is quality assurance... The effectiveness, safety, efficiency and adequacy of care, along with its acceptability to patients and the community, should be at least as important as the amount and sophistication of equipment and drugs used."

- "Target 33 discusses the necessity for national Health for All policies in each Member State, backed up by laws and regulations."

- "Target 36 concerns the planning, training and use of personnel in accordance with Health for All policies and with emphasis on primary healthcare. All health professionals should have training in teamwork, communication and primary healthcare techniques, but nurses and midwives should also develop new skills in assessment, planning, decision making, research and epidemiology."

- "The last of the Regional Targets for Health for All concerns the appropriate use of technology...providing the best care does not necessarily mean using complex machines. Some nursing personnel are already involved in testing and evaluating technology in hospitals, but they should also help determine the appropriate use of technology in primary healthcare.

What new nurses need

To fulfill such goals and to fill such a role (which looks very similar to that of a professional nurse case manager here in the USA), it seems to me that such a generalist nurse needs a university education which focuses on four integrated and integrating areas of study.

1. a solid foundation in the basic sciences,

2. a comprehensive series of courses to develop psychosocial, analytical and communication skills,

3. a thorough introduction to human values and ethics, as well as health regulation and health law, and

4. a pragmatic, hands-on internship to develop the problem-solving logic and dynamics of all of the above.

On a thoroughly pragmatic basis, today's hospitals and health organizations already are demanding (with a demand that far outstrips supplies) **nurse practitioners** (*employers*: HMOs, physicians' offices, outpatient departments, clinics, eldercare facilities, public health, business and industry, group practice IPAs, universities, and voluntary agencies), **nurse anesthetists** (*employers*: hospitals, outpatient surgeries, physician group practices, HMOs), **nurse midwives** (*employers*: hospitals, birthing centers, HMOs, physician group practices, voluntary agencies, clinics), and **critical care nurses** (*employers*: hospitals).

At the moment the largest area of demand is for critical care nurses. Moreover, with a projected increase of 30 percent in the nation's critical care beds in the next five years, the demand for critical care nurses will escalate dramatically. For the most part, these nurses need a thorough knowledge of the basic sciences, a high tech orientation, the ability to function well under stress and high capacity for flexibility and endurance. They are and must be prepared to work as team members integrating their efforts thoroughly with those of physicians, respiratory technologists, etc. Although demand is likely to tail-off in the latter half of the '90s, this role will continue to be an influencing force in nursing education and practice for the foreseeable future.

However, in the latter half of the '90s, the critical care nurses' inpatient counterpart, the adult med-surg nurse will receive more and more attention as the vast majority of inpatient beds will be adult med-surg (20% critical care, 15% swing beds, and 40% med-surg, with 5% OB, Peds, Psych, etc.). These nurses will need a thorough grounding in the basic sciences, an indepth preparation in gerontology, an interpersonal focus and an ability to work collaboratively with professional nurse case managers, physicians, and other specialists.

As surgery moves ever more rapidly to the outpatient setting, the O.R. nurse increasingly will be called upon to assess, prepare, assist and recover patients. O.R. case managers will follow high-risk patients, follow-up on patients in their homes and workplaces, and oversee service in "Recovery Care Centers." These O.R. case managers will coordinate care in both inpatient and outpatient areas.

The role of the *nurse clinical specialist* is evolving rapidly in two directions: one is toward an almost total blending with that of the nurse practitioner and the other is toward the role of the professional nurse case manager. At any rate, the clinical specialist role most likely will be submerged in the other two by the end of the '90s.

Arenas, not levels, of practice

Practice is being differentiated by necessity and by demand. Rather than *levels* of practice (i.e., "professional" versus "technical"), we must consider *arenas of practice:*

- **Arena 1:** the clinical nurse who works in hospitals or other facilities and whose principal focus is to design and deliver direct care to the majority of people who become ill, need surgery, or reside in eldercare facilities. For their complex or high-risk patients, they collaborate with nurse case managers in the design and delivery of this direct care.

- **Arena 2:** the nurse specialists who design and deliver care to patients with discrete, identifiable needs and/or who limit their practices to circumscribed areas (midwives, anesthetists, practitioners, etc.). Employed in a variety of settings, they are prepared at masters and doctoral levels.

- **Arena 3:** the nurse case manager who coordinates with primary nurses, physicians, social workers, home health nurses, etc., in the design, delivery and evaluation of care for high-risk patients in the hospital and in the community. Employed by hospitals, these nurses are prepared to baccalaureate and masters levels and most closely resemble those "nurse generalists" referred to by our European colleagues.

As these roles become more clearly delineated, the most important single political challenge for nurses will be this: NOT DEFENDING FUNCTIONS AND ROLES THAT ARE OBSOLETE. The most important single consideration will be: TO GIVE TIME AND ATTENTION TO THE EMOTIONAL AND RELATIONSHIP ASPECTS OF THE ROLE CHANGES. When roles change, so do relationships with colleagues, co-workers, and most importantly, with peers. Change always hurts, even when it's good. THE organizational imperative of the '90s will be to develop and support STRONG, COMPETENT, FIRST-LINE NURSE MANAGERS who will be energized by these changes in nurses' clinical roles. These nurse managers will coordinate the activities of all the arenas of practice and provide linkages to the organization and its resources.

We nurses are on the edge right now—we're actually redesigning ourselves—and there's no turning back.

February 1990

Touch-Tempered Technology

In his book, *In One Era and Out the Other,* Sam Levenson writes, "Man, endowed with that incredible computer known as the human brain, has used it to invent an electronic brain that will protect him from the dangers of personal involvement. Electronic impulses prevent man from acting on human impulses. Except for the fact that the information we store in the machine may already be prejudiced or obsolete, the machine is assumed to be more objective, therefore more honest than man. It cannot be sentimental (Tears rust the components)...I wonder if the synthetic, automatic, electronic world we are bequeathing to our children may not be at least partly responsible for sending them off on drug trips in search of lost senses buried, but possibly alive somewhere under layers of airproof, tasteproof, smellproof, touchproof ersatz abundance."

Of course, he was right—not so much in blaming technology as in pointing out the results of applying high tech without a counterweight of humanity. In the 1840s studies proved that infants fed artificially and essentially left untouched, literally turned their faces to the wall and died. In the 1980s, we learned that adults in intensive care units also die without human touch.

In 1982, John Naisbitt noted the parallel growth of high technologies and highly personal expressions: he claims that one balances the other. In *Megatrends,* he wrote, "Whenever new technology is introduced into society, there must be a counterbalancing human response—that is, high touch—or the technology is rejected. The more high tech, the more high touch." Certainly this seems to be the case today. Several surveys and polls conducted by the AMA, the AHA and the Institute for the Future in the latter half of the 80s revealed that:

- people are more concerned about convenience and accessibility in health services than in the past
- the public increasingly is defining "quality" in terms of health professionals' *time* and *concern*

EXHIBIT I

Technology	Human Response (Trend)	Impact on Healthcare
1. Computers and communications	Demands for more distinct and individually tailored arrangements for patients. Demands for time and concern.	Faster communication of information, bedside computerization, smart cards for patients, computerized "error prevention" programs, teleconferencing, growth of MIS.
2. Transplants, artificial organs, prosthetics	Patient's and family's insistence on participation in decision making. Growth in the "right to die" movement, possible legalization of mercy killing.	Development of rationing schemes, greater reliance on ethics committees, growth in number of ICU beds, increasing inpatient acuity and increasing shortage of nurses.
3. Surgical advances, endoscopy, lasers	Time spent before surgery in teaching and learning, people sent into the home after surgery as follow-up. Twenty-four-hour hot-lines to answer questions and give reassurance.	Increase in outpatient surgeries, growth of surgicenters, increasing preoperative role of nurses, use of professional nurse case manager to follow more complicated patients through the course of their illness.
4. Drugs, vaccines, drug delivery	Patient control of pain medication, self-administration of many drugs.	Computerized design makes it possible to tailor drugs quickly, newer drug delivery systems enable self-medication while preventing error/overdoses. Outpatient biochemical treatment of serious psychiatric disorders.
5. Home diagnostic tools	Self-administration, self-controlling, self-monitoring.	Greater sharing of information with patients, movement of some tests almost exclusively to the home, teaching patients how to use, interpret, and report the results of their own tests.
6. Magnetic Resonance Imaging and Positron Emission Tomography	Move to (and demand for) less invasive diagnostics and therapeutics—self and consumer driven.	Costs of these and other technologies in making priority decisions for purchase. Also, physician and nursing specialists will balance high-tech interventions with the healing impact of humor, positive attitudes, biofeedback, and spiritual support.
7. Genetic engineering, human gene therapy	Home care and home births are increasing in popularity. Also open-adoptions involve natural parents with their child and adoptive parents. Family and "family values" commanding more attention.	Ethical problems of abortion, use of fetal tissue, creation of life to benefit a third party, and the like force health professionals into moral choices for which they are poorly prepared.
8. Monoclonal antibodies, DNA probes	Increasing emphasis on the right to privacy and on patients' rights to refuse testing, to the full results of all tests they do consent to take, and patient determination about the dissemination of the results of tests.	MAbs fuse cancer cells with antibody-producing cells to help treat any disease entity which invokes an antibody response. Can monitor drug levels for chemotherapy and diabetic patients and hormone levels for fertility control and can deliver substances to targeted body sites. DNA probes can be used to detect infectious diseases, presence of drugs, prenatal abnormalities, and even disease susceptibility. Much more testing moved to outpatient, physician office, and home.

- patients not only want to be part of their health teams, they are seeking self-care for everything from maintaining their health to testing themselves for pregnancy.

While high tech in healthcare has brought multi-organ transplants, microsurgery and genetic engineering, recent trends move normal births into low-tech birthing centers, dying patients into hospices, and even high tech care into the home. Against this backdrop, technological trends—and their counterbalancing *human responses*—can be identified and their impact on the healthcare system in general and nursing in particular can be assured.

When the Institute for the Future queried several experts about the technologies most likely to have a major impact on healthcare, they identified the following in order of priority (see Exhibit I). Their counterbalancing human responses are found in the next column, and finally, the impact on healthcare facilities and professionals are listed in the third column.

To quote Naisbitt again: "Whenever institutions introduce new technology to customers or employees, they should build in a high touch component; if they don't, people will try to create their own or reject the new technology." The experts advise: 1. offer people *options*—don't force the technology; 2. provide plenty of people-support—don't isolate workers in cubicles no matter what efficiency engineers say: people need people to counterbalance the technology; and 3. get people involved—train and cross-train *continually*.

We cannot allow—nor will human nature allow us to allow—instinct to become extinct. We owe it to ourselves to make the best use of tools—to soften their sharp edges with human consciousness—which comes from our five senses which, in turn, don't make much sense without empathy, sympathy, love: in short, without conscience.

We need conscience to temper our technology—to add that touch which will make it strong and effective in producing human well-being. This is the trend that will—and must—dominate the future.

JULY 1990

THE EXCELLENCE WITHIN

"How can I soar with the eagles when I work with turkeys?" This lament, in one form or another, is frequently heard in nursing circles. Ordinarily, it is followed by the question: "Why doesn't management *do* something about *them*?"

Not to mix a metaphor, let's talk turkey! For the most part, "management" can't do anything about *them*. But you can. Let me explain. Management can't fire someone—or even discipline an employee—who is merely mediocre: unenthusiastic but compliant, discourteous but not quite rude, adequate but not skillful. The best of the worst and the worst of the best. So-so.

It's a real problem and, like infection, it spreads to other staff members. Ideally, management can avoid the problem by carefully selecting staff. Once hired, it's darn near next to impossible for management to get rid of someone like this. However, what management can't do, peer pressure often can. That is, peer pressure can either force them to improve or force them to get out.

If this is true in the "workplace in general"—and it is—it is doubly true for professionals in their workplaces: the collegial influence, added to the synergy (interaction of personalities) of the work group has a powerful effect.

The origins of collegiality

The concept of collegiality is thousands of years old, and most likely has its origins in that same group of Pythagorean philosophers who gave birth to the concept of "profession". Before it is anything else, the collegial relationship is a human relationship. Thus, nurses' mutual humanity—with all the limits and rights attached thereto—forms the fundamental framework for their collegial relationships. Added to this is nurses' interdependence, as well as their shared commitment to the public's health. That is, to the extent to which nurses recognize their mutual interests, build upon their common knowledge base, and acknowledge the debt they owe to their predecessors and teachers, they will offer support and guidance to their peers. Recognition of one's own capabilities and limits—even the structure of work in most facilities—leads nurses to rely on the expertise of their colleagues.

The third element of the collegial relationship, the shared experience of the practice of the profession, breathes life into it. Shared experience creates a bond, in this case, a professional bond among people. It consists of what it means, what it feels like, to practice. Nurses happen to be members of a profession which, by its very nature, brings them into contact with a great deal of human tragedy. Studies have been done on people who have witnessed a tragedy: every study shows increased stress that persists over time. Nurses not only witness the tragedies of others, they are expected to respond to them with both competence and compassion—usually in equal measure. However, there are those times when the only thing we have left to give is compassion.

The origins of excellence

Neither competence nor compassion is learned from a book. They are behaviors—characteristics of professional practice—which are demonstrated rather than taught. One sees them in action and chooses to (or not to) adopt them as one's own. In terms of the sociology of the profession, the function of the professional bond is described as that of role modeling and role internalization. But it is more than that. The shared experience which produces the bond also begets a common understanding which enables professionals to reach out and help one another in special ways.

The discovery and understanding of oneself as a professional stems from one's perception of other professionals. More precisely and powerfully, between their first experience of a professional relationship and their last, professionals actually exchange characters. One's character consists of the sum total of one's value choices. It follows, then, that one's professional character consists of the sum total of the value choices one has made in professional practice. For example, studies have shown that a nurse placed in a unit where excellent nursing is practiced soon is striving and growing to reach the level of excellence demonstrated by her *peers*. If the same nurse is placed in a unit where nursing practice is poor, most often the nurse's practice will descend to the lowest common denominator on the floor. What is at issue here is not knowledge, experience or skill, but *value* choices. Nurses affect one another so profoundly that they actually influence one another's value choices.

The function of collegiality

Nursing is a *human service*. The economists tell us that human services are produced and consumed simultaneously. It follows that nursing has its existence only in its practitioners and in their practice. To the extent that nurses support, counsel, guide and critique one another, they enhance the profession. For better or worse, each nurse creates "nursing" every day in practice. Anything which undermines the practitioner undermines the profession.

Professional relationships *enable* one to be a professional through identification with others and through finding again the dilemmas of others within oneself. Such relationships don't tell one *how to act* as much as they teach one *how to be*. The exchange of characters between self and others creates *what one is* as a nurse and, at the same time, the ideal of what a nurse should be. Consequently, the level of excellence found in practice is more a function of the collegial bond than of administrative policies.

Excellence comes from *within* the profession and *within* the staff. If staff tolerates mediocrity, practice will be mediocre. Management can create the environment, but only nurses can create nursing.

October 1990

HIV TESTING

"Jake," said his friend who had been reading in the paper of a number of fatal accidents, "if you had to choose between one or 'tother, which would you rather be in, a collision or an explosion?"

"Well," said Jake, "I guess I'd rather be in a collision."

"How come?"

"Why, if you are in a collision there you are, but if you are in an explosion where are you?"

Jake has given us a piece of homey advice that we'd do well to consider as we approach an emotional—and potentially danger-ous—question: *Should HIV testing be mandatory for healthcare workers?*

The slippery slope

Both the American Nurses Association and the American Medical Association have taken clear, unequivocal stands: *No*. Full stop. *Testing of healthcare workers (HCWs) should be voluntary, not manda-tory*. Responsible, caring professionals voluntarily seek testing when or if they fear that they could infect their patients. Any other posi-tion, they claim, leads to a "slippery slope" down which the American people will slide to the lowest levels of bigotry and cruel-ty. First (so the argument goes) there will be mandatory testing of HCWs, then patients, and then all will be reported and exposed, then all the infected will be quarantined, then all will be put in concentration-type camps to die.

Could this happen? *Yes it could*. Especially if people's fears are fanned rather than calmed. It seems to me that responsible health-care workers would *want* to calm the public's fears and, thus, pre-vent the semi-hysterical (and possibly opportunistic) posturing of politicians (e.g., Jesse Helms) who have considerable power and who could push through laws that foster—nay, demand—inhu-manity.

Of rights and privileges

Indeed, healthcare workers are human beings and citizens. They have human and legal rights, among which is the right to bodily integrity (which, presumably, is broad enough to cover a "right to refuse testing"). However, they are people who have chosen to earn their livings by dealing with the bodies and lives of other people. This is not so much a right as it is a privilege: a privilege granted by society (through subsidy and licensure) and a privilege which can be withdrawn. The notion that a HCW, *as a citizen*, can refuse HIV testing is quite defensible. However, the notion that HCWs, granted the social privilege of practice, may *refuse to take actions* which calm and protect the public—*and* continue to practice their professions—is highly debatable. Moreover, many a HCW has demanded that all patients be tested—and that all HCWs involved in their care be appraised of the results of the patients' tests—so that they can protect themselves. Certainly, adherence to *universal* precautions ought to be enough. And, surely, any health professional *ought to know* that the undiagnosed patient, especially one who falls into the "low risk" categories, presents the greatest danger of transmission. And yet, nonetheless, literally thousands of healthcare workers believe they have a right to know the patients' HIV status—which demand, by its very nature, includes mandatory testing and mandatory disclosure, at least to the healthcare team.

> **Universal testing of *all* healthcare workers is even more expensive than it is impractical.**

For years, drivers have been licensed. Driving is a social privilege, even if one earns one's living that way (e.g., truck and taxi-cab drivers). If a police officer suspects that a driver has been drinking, he can demand that the driver be tested. Drivers have the right to refuse the test, but if they do, they will lose their licenses to drive. And so far, the country hasn't gone to the dogs: this practice even seems to improve matters for most people.

Testing healthcare professionals could be handled in the same way. However, there should be some modification.

1. Universal testing of *all* healthcare workers is even more expensive than it is impractical.

2. Therefore, testing should be limited to those healthcare workers who participate in high-risk, exposure-prone procedures. The Centers for Disease Control (CDC) defines such procedures as follows:

"Characteristics of exposure-prone procedures include digital palpation of a needle tip in a body cavity or the simultaneous presence of the HCW's fingers and a needle or other sharp instrument or object in a poorly visualized or highly confined anatomic site. Performance of exposure-prone procedures presents a recognized risk of percutaneous injury to the HCW, and—if such an injury occurs—the HCW's blood is likely to contact the patient's body cavity, subcutaneous tissues, and/or mucous membranes."

3. Patients who are to undergo high-risk, invasive and/or exposure-prone procedures, also should be tested.

4. There should be frequent retesting of those HCWs whose practice requires participation in exposure-prone, high-risk, invasive procedures.

5. HCWs who are HIV positive or who become HIV positive, have a right to privacy, but they have no right to expose others to risk. Therefore, they must not participate in exposure-prone procedures.

6. All involved, patients and personnel, should know that HIV testing is not always accurate, i.e., people can test negative for several months after they have been infected.

Before we go any further

The Centers for Disease Control issued guidelines in a pamphlet entitled "Recommendations for Preventing Transmission of Human Immunodeficiency Virus and Hepatitis B. Virus to Patients During Exposure-Prone Procedures." In this document, the CDC unequivocally states:

"The recommendations outlined in this document are based on the following considerations:

- Infected HCWs who adhere to universal precautions and who do not perform invasive procedures pose no risk for transmitting HIV or HBV to patients.

- Infected HCWs who adhere to universal precautions and who perform certain exposure-prone procedures pose a small risk for transmitting HBV to patients.

- HIV is transmitted much less readily than HBV."

At this time, the CDC recommends:

- "All HCWs should adhere to universal precautions, including the appropriate use of hand washing, protective barriers, and care in the use and disposal of needles and other sharp instruments. HCWs who have exudative lesions or weeping dermatitis should refrain from all direct patient care and from handling patient-care equipment and devices used in performing invasive procedures until the condition resolves. HCWs should also comply with current guidelines for disinfection and sterilization of reusable devices used in invasive procedures.

- "Currently available data provide no basis for recommendations to restrict the practice of HCWs infected with HIV or HBV who perform invasive procedures not identified as exposure-prone, provided the infected HCWs practice recommended surgical or dental technique and comply with universal precautions and current recommendations for sterilization/disinfection.

- "Exposure-prone procedures should be identified by medical/surgical/dental organizations and institutions at which the procedures are performed.

- "HCWs who perform exposure-prone procedures should know their HIV antibody status. HCWs who perform exposure-prone procedures and who do not have serologic evidence of immunity to HBV from vaccination or from previous infection should know their HBsAg status and, if that is positive, should also know their HBeAg status.

• "HCWs who are infected with HIV or HBV (and are HBeAg positive) should not perform exposure-prone procedures unless they have sought counsel from an expert review panel and been advised under what circumstances, if any, they may continue to perform these procedures. Such circumstances would include notifying prospective patients of the HCW's seropositivity before they undergo exposure-prone invasive procedures.

• "Mandatory testing of HCWs for HIV antibody, HBsAg, or HBeAg is not recommended. The current assessment of the risk that infected HCWs will transmit HIV or HBV to patients during exposure-prone procedures does not support the diversion of resources that would be required to implement mandatory testing programs. Compliance by HCWs with recommendations can be increased through education, training, and appropriate confidentiality safeguards."

The CDC needs:

• "Clearer definition of the nature, frequency, and circumstances of blood contact between patients and HCWs during invasive procedures.

• Development and evaluation of new devices, protective barriers and techniques that may prevent such blood contact without adversely affecting the quality of patient care.

• More information on the potential for HIV and HBV transmission through contaminated instruments.

• Improvements in sterilization and disinfection techniques for certain reusable equipment and devices.

• Identification of factors that may influence the likelihood of HIV or HBV transmission after exposure to HIV- or HBV-infected blood."

Professionals and their associations should place high priority on meeting these needs. Once definitions are clearer and more complete, healthcare workers who participate in professionally defined, high-risk, exposure-prone procedures should be tested. If they refuse, they should not—by administrative policy, one hopes, rather than law—participate in activities which could put patients at risk. No one, homosexual or heterosexual, health professional or patient, wants to contract a fatal disease.

It seems to be far preferable to deal with this "collision of rights" rather than an explosion of fear and bigotry.

As 'Jake' would say, "There we are," flattened and battered but at least we know where we are. Jesse Helms' proposed law, i.e., that HIV positive HCWs who knowingly participate in high-risk, exposure-prone procedures go to jail for 10 years, has lit the fuse. If the explosion occurs, then "where are we?"

September 1991

FREE THE HOSPICE 6

Six Montana nurses must stand trial—not for malpractice but rather for malfeasance. Their "crime"? They are accused of hoarding narcotics to give to home-bound hospice patients whose prescriptions run out at inconvenient times. Like the middle of the night when physicians are asleep and pharmacies are closed.

These nurses, all of whom work for St. Christopher's Hospice, allegedly asked the families of recently deceased patients to donate any unused painkillers. This, presumably, is how they accumulated the stockpile with which they helped living patients who used up their medications too soon.

...the source may have been unorthodox...

To my knowledge, no one has accused the nurses of giving any patient an overdose. If they are guilty of anything, they are "guilty" of an act of mercy...But this "act" would have nothing to do with mercy killing, although it certainly would have a great deal to do with quality of life. Indeed, there is no evidence that the "Hospice 6" did anything other than "give the right patient, the right drug, in the right amount, by the right route, and (most certainly) at the right time." Exactly as nurses have been taught to do for the last hundred years or so...even if the source of the drugs might have been a bit unorthodox...

...and authorities may disagree...

Now heaven knows that most state boards tend to be *very* conservative in their interpretations of nursing law. Yet, having investigated this incident, Montana's State Board of Nursing recommended that the nurses be "counseled". Nothing more. However, a zealous (and politically ambitious?) prosecutor decided to press charges anyway. He is demanding that these nurses be punished "to the fullest extent of the law."

...but have you ever seen early morning pain?

Obviously, in the world as we find it, ignorance, rigidity and power are a dangerous mix. One wonders if this prosecutor has ever seen pain (searing, grinding, soul-wrenching pain) at three in the morning? Has he ever heard the desperation in a man's voice as he pleads for help for someone he loves? Does he know anything about the fear that comes from the anticipation of pain and loss of control over pain? Ignorance is a dangerous thing.

...the letter of the law...

The State Board of Nursing, duly instituted to interpret the Nursing Practice Statute and to protect the public from incompetence or abuse, found the nurses innocent of any wrong-doing. They were imprudent. That's it. They are to be counseled to be prudent. So be it. However, this prosecutor holds that the letter, if not the spirit, of the law has been broken. This apparently is a grievous fault...and grievously must the nurses answer it. Rigidity is a dangerous thing.

...the power and the duty...

A lawyer, a prosecutor, an officer of the court has both the duty and the power to uphold the law. However, unbending adherence to duty is a frightening thing. And power wielded without compassion becomes brute force. In the United States of America, we claim that we have a nation "by the people, for the people and of the people." The people of Montana are speaking out: they are carrying placards that read "Free the Hospice 6" and putting bumper stickers that say the same thing on their cars. Law should not strain the "quality of mercy"...

> **Power wielded without compassion becomes brute force.**

...to protect the truly vulnerable...

We do have reason to fear lest the law be changed inappropriately and those who need its protection be left unguarded. Several weeks ago I traveled to Minnesota to take part in a seminar sponsored by the American Cancer Society. In the afternoon, we had a panel discussion which dealt with ethical problems in the care of cancer patients. One panelist, a philosopher who is a member of the Hemlock Society, held that thousands of nurses and doctors are deliberately killing people with overdoses to relieve them of the misery of

> **We do not need a law to protect us so that we *can* kill people.**

intractable pain. He argued that the law must be changed to legalize these efforts and protect those who kill out of mercy. Indeed, legislation which would permit mercy killing is on the ballot in the state of Washington, and the Hemlock Society has initiated steps for referenda in three other states. Initially, any change in the law would be limited to those conscious, rational adults who ask to be put to death. However, such beneficence should not be limited, so the reasoning goes, only to the competent.

...invalid suppositions...

To my mind, this man from the Hemlock Society seemed to be operating on suppositions which "ain't necessarily so." For example, the notion that thousands of doctors and nurses are deliberately killing for mercy. On what basis is such an outrageous claim made? In my own experience (which, I assure you, is far more extensive than that of the Hemlockian), both physicians and nurses tend to exercise every effort to try to keep people alive—sometimes for far too long. We are not killing people (at least not on purpose) and we do not need a law to protect us so that we *can* kill people (with or without their consent?).

Laws are written to protect all the people, but especially those who are most vulnerable...and who could be more vulnerable than those who cannot speak for themselves? The Hemlockians also presuppose that thousands of people are experiencing *intractable* pain. If so, it is because they are being mismanaged medically—or, possibly, because prosecutors in some jurisdictions make no exceptions to the general rule, interpret laws without regard for the context of a situation, and apply their power with brute force...and seek to punish any infraction, however minor, "to the fullest extent of the law." Power is a dangerous thing in such hands.

Ignorance, rigidity and power—a dangerous mix in today's world. Dangerous for those who act out of compassion, dangerous for those who are most vulnerable, and ultimately dangerous for society which learns, in just such manner, to disrespect the law.

Free the Hospice 6—for their sake, for nursing's sake, and for the peoples' sake.

July 1991

ADVANCED LICENSURE: PERSONAL PLUM OR PUBLIC SHIELD?

The rhetoric is awesome: back-stepping, word-eating, wonderful... From many of those organizations which endorsed baccalaureate education into practice... From many of those dedicated people preaching lifelong education for nurses... From many of those painstaking purveyors of differentiated practice.

Well, the National Council of State Boards of Nursing (NCSBN) called their bluff. At their national meeting, NCSBN will consider recommending model legislation that, among other things, would institute (if adopted by each state) advanced licensure by examination and require a nurse to have earned a masters degree in clinical nursing to sit for the advanced practice licensure exam. NCSBN officials quite correctly sent a copy of this proposal, *in advance*, to all the nursing specialty groups for comment, and to the American Nurses Association (ANA), which promptly sent copies to all its Constituents.

Exit: glorious visions of educational status and professional growth. **Enter:** pragmatism wrapped in high-toned rationalization.

The ANA House of Delegates voted overwhelmingly to oppose NCSBN's proposal—a move that should surprise no one—and endorsed the notion that "the profession" will regulate itself, presumably through certification. The problem is that the profession has no way to regulate itself. Certification is offered by a large number of organizations (including ANA), efforts to establish an independent credentialing center to credential the credentialers has not met with success, requirements to take the exams vary, and one is led to believe the validity of some of these exams can best be described as hit or miss.

Nursing's response to this splendid opportunity to protect the public and advance its best and brightest is curious. To paraphrase a child's nursery rhyme:

"Little Nurse Horner sat in the corner
Eating her practice pie
NCSBN put in its thumb
And pulled out a plum
And frightened Nurse Horner away!"

Heaven forbid that advanced practitioners be legitimized: it could mean control...some states are too restrictive...it's a plot to oppress nurses or divide them or...they might think they're special. This latter argument—i.e., that advanced practice registered nurses will think they are "special" (so that means we shouldn't let them come into existence?)—smacks of anti-intellectualism. A nurse is a nurse is a nurse...any nurse who learns more or does more or stands out is "out of place," arrogant and presuming. Instead of the "caring" profession, nursing is becoming known as the homogenized profession.

> **Heaven forbid that advanced practitioners be legitimized: it could mean control...it's a plot to oppress nurses or divide them or... they might think they're special.**

The problem is, of course, that none of the organizations, ANA included, have the legal authority to expand or limit advanced practice. The NCSBN doesn't either. Such authority is vested in each individual state. The National Council (NCSBN) can adopt model legislation which individual state boards may choose to recommend to their state's legislature. The ensuing political process allows for considerable adjustment before enactment.

The reason a state requires licensure is *to protect the public* from incompetents and quacks. Secondarily (and usually quite happily for the licensee), licensure *legitimates* practice by granting it public recognition and sanction. Rightly or wrongly, it also carves out an area that becomes the license holders' exclusive preserves.

This redounds to the profession's welfare. It grants status and privilege. With these, practitioners' incomes rise—a real plum indeed.

Libertarian concerns

This latter observation frets some libertarians who claim that licensure limits the people's access to a service and creates a legally privileged class. Firmly convinced that people can and should protect themselves, they advocate the abolition of all licenses. Government's role is *laissez-faire*. If the people aren't smart enough to protect themselves, then *c'est la vie!*

Lawyers cant

One objection to advanced licensure, i.e., that there is no proof that nurses engaged in advanced practice who don't have masters degrees (or for that matter, baccalaureate degrees) have caused serious harm to patients—more or less reflects this view.

Let us grant that long years of experience and on-the-job training may render them competent. Amending this model legislation to provide for "grandfathering" by examination would solve this problem. Surely a competent practitioner need not fear an examination. Particularly when taking an exam could weed out incompetents *before* they endanger the public and damage the hard-won credibility of the advanced practice nurse.

Remember all those nurses and nursing leaders who urged us to be PROACTIVE rather than REACTIVE? I know lawyers say in court *"Prove* that this person has harmed someone," but I thought professionals were proactive. Wouldn't a professional want to prevent harm when possible?

Reduced access...

Another objection rests on the claim that we already have many nurses engaged in advanced practice without masters degrees and without advanced licensure. If they are prevented from practicing, it will limit people's access to care. True...but the supply need not be unduly limited if nurses engaged in advanced practice (with or without masters degrees) prior to the passage of the legislation sit for the exam. If they pass, they can practice. If they cannot, perhaps they should not be engaged in advanced practice.

What is really behind all this? At least 35 states have granted prescriptive authority to advanced practice nurses and the rest are likely to follow. Subsequently, each state legislated access to advanced practice and prescriptive privileges in various ways. Some require licensure. Others do not. Some require that a physician approve the nurses' "prescriptions." Others do not. Some limit nurses' prescriptive authority to one list of drugs. Others set a different list. Still others are far less restrictive. But all of them intend—as they must—to protect their citizens as they see best. Unfortunately, the results are disorderly. A uniform approach would bring order and consistency to a chaotic situation.

The problem with the proposal

Unfortunately, NCSBN's proposal "clumps" specialty and advanced practice nurses together. To confound matters further, the profession seems to be equating certification with advanced practice. I suggest that it is not.

Certification recognizes excellence in an area of practice, but it does not expand its boundaries.

Advance practice takes nurses beyond the bounds of nursing as it is commonly practiced. While all nurses need the freedom to make decisions about nursing care, advanced practice nurses need that freedom *and more* because they make decisions about matters not included in generic practice, only one example of which is prescribing drugs. While all nurses design and provide nursing services and carry out the medical regimen, advanced practice nurses not only design and provide nursing services but also *integrate* what used to be considered medical practices into those nursing services.

On the other hand, highly specialized nurses, e.g., nurse anesthetists and nurse midwives, have focused both their education and practice in *one* narrowly defined area. At the very least, they graduate from a generic nursing program, sit for generic licensure and then return to a very specific school in which they develop very specific skills that prepare them to provide highly specialized services. Once graduated from their intensive, skill-specific courses, they sit for a certification exam and then apply for a *separate* license to practice their specific skills. In some states, the Board of Medicine, rather than the Board of Nursing grants this license. Such special licenses authorize the nurses who hold them to perform specific tasks other nurses are not legally allowed to perform. Many specialized nurses have masters degrees in their specific, clearly defined arenas. Many do not...yet.

Conceptualize practice as it is...

Perhaps nursing would object less if State Boards of Nursing could conceptualize the nursing profession differently. For example, nursing practice itself could be described in terms of arenas of practice:

• **Arena I: Generic Practice.** This arena includes all RNs working in every area of practice in institutions and agencies throughout the country. The requirements of entry are, minimally, an ADN plus generic licensure. These nurses staff all the units and areas of practice. Each state's generic nurse practice act describes and circumscribes their practice. Certification recognizes excellence in the specific areas of practice.

• **Arena II: Highly Specialized Practice.** This arena encompasses nurses whose limited and specialized practice has been clearly defined by its entry requirements. Minimally, such nurses must graduate from a generic nursing program, earn generic licensure, graduate from a specialty-specific school, and achieve separate licensure as, viz., nurse anesthetists or nurse midwives. They may perform all actions and services provided by generic nurses, plus the specific skills encompassed by their additional, separate license. Usually, but not always, highly specialized nurses limit their practice to their specific field of expertise.

- **Arena III: Advanced Practice.** Advanced practice nurses are noted both for their broad preparation and for the broad scope of their activities. *Today,* the requirements to become a nurse practitioner, a clinical nurse specialist, or a nurse psychotherapist are clear: BSN, generic licensure, a clinical masters degree in nursing and, in some states, other credentialing mechanisms. If the NCSBN proposal is accepted, provisions should be made for grandfathering *by examination* all nurses currently filling "advanced practitioner" roles, e.g., nurse practitioners, clinical nurse specialists, nurse psychotherapists.

- **Arena IV: Functional Practice.** This arena includes nurses who perform functions for and within the profession, primarily nurse administrators and nurse educators. Other functional roles include nurse epidemiologist, nurse researcher, and nurse consultant. Even nurse editors belong in this category. Although professional organizations do have significant influence on developing criteria for such positions, employing institutions largely determine their distinguishing characteristics by the position requirements they set. They must, of course, be graduates of a generic program in nursing and holders of a generic license. Advanced degrees almost always are necessary. Advanced licensure is not. In some instances, certification recognizes excellence in practice.

Let us all, in every area and arena of practice, *help* the NCSBN create the best possible advanced practice act. Let every nursing organization turn its considerable talents to ironing out the kinks in the NCSBN proposal. That is true self-governance. Demands for "control of practice," in the absence of visible mechanisms for exercising such self control, are geared only to nurses' convenience. To leave the people unprotected—and demand proof of malfeasance before we act—is directly contrary to every value nurses have espoused in the last 30 years: education, accountability, patient advocacy, differentiated practice.

August 1992

PERSONALIZED CARE IN A STANDARDIZED WORLD

One Sunday morning an elderly woman approached a prominent Bishop after church and gushed enthusiastically, "Bishop, you'll never know what your sermon meant to me. It was just like water to a drowning man!"

Less enthusiastically, many nurses and physicians hold exactly the same sentiment about the practice guidelines which the Agency for Health Care Policy and Research (AHCPR) is generating these days. Already flooded with standards from such diverse sources as their professional associations, the JCAHO, private and public payors, state and federal government, consumer groups and hospitals, like water to a drowning man, they are now inundated with yet another tidal wave of "guidance" from a well-intentioned source.

Of guidelines and standards

Physicians in particular decry the dehumanization of the profession by all such "cookbook" medicine. And nurses join them in wringing their hands over the institutionalized emphasis on costs, labor efficiencies, and decreasing lengths of stay which speed the process. Indeed, the cynics among us believe that saving money, not lives is the current "hidden agenda" behind the promulgation of practice guidelines.

Nevertheless, whether cynic or optimist, we would be hard put to make a convincing case against establishing respectable standards. Who **wants** to support substandard care? And who **could afford** suprastandard care?

"Ah!" we retort, "Just **whose** standards are we actually getting?"

The answer, for better or worse is "ours." Panels of experts gathered from every specialty are formulating them. How are they selected? Professional reputation, publication and the like do influence choices, but the recommendations solicited from nursing and medical organizations usually are acted upon.

The problem does not really arise from who sets the standards or even how they are set. It doesn't even lie in how much clout is attached to practice guidelines by, for instance, attaching reimbursement to adherence. Rather, the very presumption that standardizing necessarily means depersonalizing is the heart of the matter. While guidelines may standardize **regimens, interactions** remain very personal indeed.

Of people and relationships

The humanity of the patient is at the core of the service he or she needs. Thus, the clinical care of the patient comprises only one aspect of care—and often not even the most important one. The professional relationship's very foundation **is** the mutual humanity of its participants; that is, each patient's human needs and each professional's response to them determine the form that relationship takes. Upon this simple foundation, patient and professional structure the particular characteristics of their relationship in any given encounter, e.g., child and parent, client and counselor, student and teacher, friend and friend, colleague and colleague and so forth, through the range of possibilities. Moreover, the structure of the professional relationship changes as the patient's needs change.

To begin even to comprehend human relationships in the professional context, we must understand that disease: 1) magnifies universal human needs, 2) generates special needs, and 3) renders the patient far more vulnerable. Therefore, health professionals not only must identify the specific physiologic damage caused by disease or trauma, but also discover the extent to which illness has wounded the patient's integrity. For the wounds of the spirit penetrate far beyond physical manifestations to the existential depths of a person's being.

The wounds of the spirit

It is true enough that different people exhibit different reactions to the threats posed by illness. Nevertheless, identifying some of these wounds calls for an examination of those factors which threaten the human spirit.

- *First of all, I lose my sense of personal independence. Illness infringes upon my autonomy. At the very least, to access any kind of care, I must go to another person, place myself before this person, reveal my deficiency or defect, and ask for help. Blatantly, disease turns an independent individual into a beggar: a position that challenges my sense of controlling my world and of being self-sufficient within it. On top of this, the more personal the disclosure, or the more threatening the disclosure, the more difficult it is likely to be for me to reveal it.*

If health professionals are sensitive to the painful humiliation which seeking care may impose, they can take the right steps to mitigate these demeaning effects. If we keep constantly in mind that we, too, are vulnerable human beings, we will reach out to each patient with friendliness and compassion.

> **If we keep constantly in mind that we, too, are vulnerable human beings, we will reach out to each patient with friendliness and compassion.**

- *Secondly, illness deprives me of my freedom of action. When I am ill, I cannot command my body to do what I want it to do. I am a bodily creature, but I use my body for more than fulfilling physiological needs and instinctual drives. I transcend such considerations to use my body to express my hopes and dreams, and to bear witness to my ideals and values.*

Losing any kind of freedom of action—locomotive, verbal, sometimes intellectual—significantly damages any patient's spirit, sometimes very seriously. Because this sense of loss is so compelling, caregivers must do everything we can to honor our patients' desire for activity and self-expression.

The responsibilities of the relationship

Very clearly, in this relationship, the patient is agonizingly vulnerable. One patient may be completely unable to hear, to see, to grasp, or to understand. Others may suffer just some degree of such physical impairments. These deficiencies are obvious and at the surface. However, the patient's value structure is not so easily ascertained. Caregivers may have to rely upon surrogates who are not always advocates, namely family members and acquaintances, to explicate a patient's value system.

Health professionals must be fully aware of the unconscious pressures which may influence surrogates whenever a patient's continued life will be burdensome. I do not mean to condemn anyone by this statement. Rather, I mean to emphasize that health professionals have a distinct responsibility to assure that any surrogates—any proxies—are, indeed, **advocates** for that patient.

In all circumstances, caregivers must be perceptive about what it is that the surrogates are saying about the patient. Sometimes, health professionals may have to assert their own value systems to fulfill this obligation. Situations in which a patient's rational capacities are damaged, and may never be retrieved, are very difficult. They place onerous burdens upon everyone—family, health professionals and society—and these complex problems do not lend themselves to easy or unilateral resolutions.

Making critical distinctions and weighing facts and values are essential to deciding satisfactory courses of action. Pain, shock, trauma and drugs all undermine my functional capacity to make choices. So does the pain imposed by the loss of wholeness and the ability to act. Thus, disease can interfere with my ability—not my right—to make decisions.

The high technology and moral pluralism of contemporary society have greatly magnified the value conflicts which complicate vital healthcare decisions. Therefore, the responsibility to respect the patient's value system has assumed vastly increased significance.

Professionals are inclined to consider "rational" only those decisions that agree with their own. However, if we are sensitive to this tendency, we are more likely to try to discover and to act upon the patient's value system rather than our own or even the family's.

The power of interaction

The corollary of these factors is that disease places the patient in the power of others. Many social as well as political institutions exercise great power over people but, once recognized, these powers can be surrounded with legal safeguards. For example, we now recognize that consent obtained under duress is not legally binding. Illness imposes threats of suffering and death that are more coercive than most things in life, yet what legal advocate or state laws can protect us from these?

Because the state cannot defend us, those persons regarded as capable of relieving such threats exercise enormous power over those in physical or psychological distress. Generally speaking, patients lack the knowledge to define the threat and they do not have the competence to reduce it. Therefore, they must depend on health professionals for both.

Whether health professionals want it or not, whether we like it or not, we do possess enormous power over those whom we serve. To deny that power establishes a situation in which, by simply refusing to admit the power we have, we can use it as we will.

Only if we acknowledge this power will we take steps to mitigate the threat it imposes. Obviously, sharing this power involves providing information for patients and their families. However, **how** they are told and **when** they are told is at least as significant as **what** they are told. Today, largely responding to fears of litigation, professionals may literally tyrannize patients with technical information. More to hedge against malpractice than to respect human rights, we overload the patient with a tremendous burden of incomprehensible information—usually in one short session. People would benefit much more from small bits of information presented in common terms when the person is ready for it and as he or she asks for it.

Avoiding depersonalization

If we do not address the existential wounds which illness causes, these wounds fester. People are defined in terms of their value choices. *Circumstances, coupled with insensitivity, force changes which my whole being rejects. Just as my body may reject a transplanted organ, so my spirit may reject values alien to it. When that happens I lose my will to live. Insofar as my values are ignored and replaced with those of other people, I lose my distinctive place in this world, indeed, my vision of who I am.*

> **However standardized the world of guidelines and critical pathways, care of the human beings within them is still intensely personal.**

Standards and guidelines deal with "how" the patient shall live, but "why" a patient chooses to live is intensely personal. Sensitivity to the patient's humanity helps professionals look beneath the surface for the human responses to actual or potential health problems.

Healing the **body** is a function of professional knowledge and skill which a practice guideline can capture. Healing the **spirit** is a function of the relationship between professional and patient which cannot be standardized. Healing a human being requires *both*. However standardized the world of guidelines and critical pathways, care of the human beings within them is still intensely personal.

October 1992

REAL NURSES DON'T WHINE

Sometime ago, I found myself a captive at a no-frills conference of nurse theorists, researchers and graduate students. These worthies cared a lot about the theoretical foundations of nursing practice, but not at all about saunas or shopping. I hate to make generalizations, but there is an inverse correlation between smart people and concern for creature comforts.

Abstraction to distraction

Day after day the conference droned on from database to conceptual framework as speaker after speaker explicated in excruciating detail nursing phenomena in language only the initiated understood. We viewed pictures of slinkies and watched, in bemused bafflement, illustrations of theories that resembled nothing so much as thousand legged worms.

Night after night, I joined the group in the hotel's small seminar rooms to listen to lectures, to watch slides, and to make notes on what we were to cover the next day. No one suspected that, in college, responding to the question, "Define a biopsychosocial need," I had written, "chocolate."

This was not a crowd interested in such disingenuous frivolity. They were *purists* who had come to this seminar to *advance nursing science*. If they had known where I was coming from, they would have been shocked. They even talked *phenomenology* before breakfast!

I wouldn't have minded (too much, at any rate) wading through hours of mind-numbing jargon in the company of earnest scholars if there had been a Nieman-Marcus on the horizon. There was not. After landing at the airport, we had been transported by bus for two hours into the country-side. Try as I might, I couldn't even find a Wal-Mart.

Listening to speeches read word for word from doctoral theses would have been bearable if, at least at the end I could have looked forward to a little bottle of wine and some munchies. Our hotel was situated in the precise center of a dry county.

There are few meetings held in parts of the world where you really have to fight to spend your money. You show me a nurses' convention and I'll show you a shopping mall. But, after three days, I gave up. I took my credit cards out of my bra and returned them to my wallet.

Meanwhile, the conference crawled along a treadmill to oblivion with stop-offs at boredom and monotony. I fantasized about sedating a speaker with a dart gun from the back row. In my day dreams I became the Queen of Hearts shouting "Off with their empirical heads." I knew I really was hallucinating when I became Meryl Streep between the sheets with Robert Redford.

Something snapped. The next day, I refused to come out of my room until the conference coordinator (I was supposed to give the closing address) pounded on my door and shouted, "Leah, stop *whining*. Real nurses can take a lot more than this."

"Venting" to "vision"

"Oh yeah," I thought. "Real nurses shop...and they never, never talk theory before coffee in the morning."

Come to think of it, real nurses don't even know there is a controversy between phenomenologists and empiricists. Real nurses don't deal with phenomena, they take care of patients. They don't worry about empiricism and they don't split philosophical hairs.

They do worry about giving someone the wrong medication.

Real nurses use disposable needles. And carry at least 690 patients.

I was on a roll now! Real nurses do not need calculators. Real nurses do not fear doctors. Real nurses do not blame anonymous "others" for their problems and they do not go about mumbling that they feel "powerless." What real nurses do on their days off is sleep.

Real nurses do not spend hours illustrating a conceptual framework. They do not speak or write in polysyllabic circumlocutions.

Real nurses do not fret about transcultural experiences: they worry about paying off their *Visa* bills.

Contrary to popular belief, real nurses *do* read. They read spreadsheets, they read patient charts, they read clinical and pharmaceutical updates, they read anything written by Judith Kranz.

Real nurses are not overachievers: they really *are* that smart.

Real nurses are not congenitally late for work.

Real nurses aren't co-dependent: they can take care of themselves while they take care of others. They are not too busy to listen to a frightened family member.

Real nurses are not afraid to cry.

A real nurse is proud of the profession and never says "I'm just a nurse."

A real nurse learns how the system works—if only out of self-protection.

A real nurse doesn't think that "tough, rational, performance-oriented, competent and no-nonsense" are accolades which apply only to men.

A real nurse *will* go to an insanely boring six-hour lecture—but only if she gets CEUs.

The one true principle

For decades, nurses have looked to science for vision and answers. They have expected scholars to rationalize and justify and professionalize nursing practice. Why can't we develop a meta theory? How did nurses ever practice without supporting data? Why am I stuck working the night shift every Christmas when I have more seniority than 99 percent of the rest of the staff and I have perfect attendance and I always document accurately and completely on every patient chart?

Monads, diads, triads, deficits, magnetic energy fields—we search endlessly for understanding.

Quantum physics, the wellness continuum, the scientific method, nursing diagnosis, advocacy, co-dependence, the uncertainty principle, the wounded inner child—we try to resolve our place in the universe.

Rogers, Neuman, Roy, King, Orem, Peplau, Major Margaret Houlihan—the greatest minds in nursing have peered into the chaos, looking for order.

Yet real nurses have always known the answer.

In their heart of hearts, they have known the one guiding principle that governs everything: *Patients will be sick 24 hours a day, 7 days a week, 365 days a year. Including weekends, nights and holidays.*

Fantasy to reality

Close your eyes.

Picture a glorious mauve and peach office. The picture window frames a distant view of the ocean; deep carpets muffle any noise.

As you turn around, you see a nurse sitting behind a 12-foot mahogany desk. She is about 30. Her hair is pulled back in a chic chignon. She's wearing a $1200 Liz Clairbourne suit, three-inch heels and sculpted nails. A telephone glued to her left ear, she is negotiating a contract for a seminar on the latest modifications of an adjusted-needs theory based upon intentionally-directed, energy-wave patterns as applied to self-help deficits among pregnant women in the final stages of labor on the third day after a full moon.

Open your eyes. *This is not a real nurse.*

Now, erase that picture from your mind.

Think about a hospital unit. It is Christmas Eve. Decorations hang limply on the walls. In the middle of this snowy night, a respirator wheezes oxygen in and out of a 24-year-old who almost succeeded in killing himself. Lights flash red and green on the monitors over the bed of an elderly woman in congestive heart failure.

How do you spot the real nurses?

They are the ones in rumpled lab coats, leaning over the side rails, trying to negotiate the only "contract" that really matters: person to person.

My reverie ended there. The Conference Coordinator was still pounding on my door. I girded my loins to face another day.

She is right you know.

Real nurses don't whine.

December 1992

THE HEART OF PATIENT CARE

I am a nurse. A professional nurse. In fact, I've devoted the lion's share of my adult life to this profession. Unlike some, I do not resent nursing: I love it. Unlike some, I do not think I could have made a better living some other way: I think there is no better job—at least not for me. Making a living is not only about *generating income*, it also has to do with making a contribution, feeling worthwhile, and finding meaning in one's work. Unlike some, I am not frustrated by the profession's "lack of progress": I know just how far nurses have come in the last 30 years.

I also know that the way we were was a good way to be. And the way we are now, is even better. But *the way we are going to be* will be the best so far. This, however, is not to say that the road ahead is going to be easy.

A wise woman's parable for today's nurse

In her book, *Wouldn't take Nothing for my Journey Now*, Maya Angelou tells the story of a poor, black woman around the turn of the century.

Unhappily married with two toddlers, the late Mrs. Annie Johnson of Arkansas "...looked up the road I was going and back the way I come, and since I wasn't satisfied, I decided to step off the road and cut me a new path." After separating from her husband, she took stock of her prospects. Barely literate, she was, nonetheless, healthy and intelligent—and she did not want her children to be reared by strangers.

There were two factories in Annie Johnson's hometown—a cotton gin and a lumber mill—but neither of them would hire a woman. So she devised a plan: since she couldn't work for the factories she'd figure out a way to make the factories work for her. She knew she wasn't much of a cook, but she could "mix groceries well enough to scare hungry from a starving man." So she used what money she had to buy groceries and spent the night making meat pies. The next day, she went to the cotton gin, and just as the lunch whistle blew, she started frying the pies. Unable to resist their delicious smell, the men bought them at a nickel apiece. She took what they didn't eat and walked five miles to the lumber mill and sold the cold meat pies to its workers for three cents. Every other day, she switched so that each set of workers got a chance to buy the fresh, hot pies. For the next few years, no matter what the weather, Annie was there with meat pies for the workers.

"When she felt certain that they had become dependent on her, she built a stall between the two hives of industry and let the men run to her for their lunchtime provisions." She was so successful that eventually her stall became a restaurant and her restaurant expanded into a store. She stepped from the road that seemed ordained for her and "cut herself a brand new path."

Maya Angelou concludes that "Each of us has a right and responsibility to assess the roads which lie ahead...and if the future road looks ominous or unpromising, then we need to gather our resolve and, carrying only the necessary baggage, step off that road into another direction. If the new choice is also unpalatable, without embarrassment, we must be ready to change that as well."

Just as Annie Johnson did, nurses—if they would succeed, if they would further their profession—must honestly and carefully take stock of their situation: what we have to offer; what deficits we must accept or correct; what obstacles we must overcome, or find a way around.

What we have to offer

Ever since Florence Nightingale wrote those fateful words, "What the nurse has to do is put the patient in the best frame possible for nature to act upon him," nurses have struggled to explain precisely what they actually do to achieve this (in contemporary parlance, "to diagnose and treat human responses to actual or potential health problems.").

In their ingenuity, nurses have managed to generate a baker's dozen of theories which purportedly "explain all"—only they don't, or they won't, or they can't, or at any rate they haven't. So, ever since one of nursing's earliest theorists, Virginia Henderson, wrote "The nurse does for the patient what the patient would do for himself, unaided, if he could," nurses have sought ways to claim their practice and lay claim to its outcomes—an infection that did not occur, a nutritional status that was not compromised, a pressure ulcer prevented, a patient who did comply with the medical regimen, patients and families who learned self-care, diseases that did not spread, and on and on...

What nurses contribute seems as obvious as it is difficult to measure and differentiate from the patients' contributions, the physicians' contributions, and society's contributions. However, in today's "outcome driven" world, it seems that nurses must at least try to disaggregate their contributions and the outcomes of their interventions.

Some obstacles to overcome

As some, but by no means all, hospitals seek to restructure themselves and redesign jobs, nurses increasingly are challenged to justify their existence. If, for example, as Henderson said, "the nurse does for the patient what the patient could do for himself" why does it take years of education to do it? If you can teach a patient to care for himself or a family member to care for the patient, why must a highly-skilled and (comparatively) highly-paid nurse have to do it while the patient is in the hospital? If you can teach a family member to do it, then you can teach a nursing assistant (multi-skilled worker, unlicensed assistive person, etc.) how to do it.

Let's take these questions one at a time.

1. It takes considerable knowledge to understand the thousands of diseases and traumas that may afflict untold numbers of human beings. It takes even more to learn what nursing interventions may be helpful at various points in the patient's recovery. It also takes judgment and perspicacity to integrate the nursing care of the patient with the medical regimen. Moreover, the more complicated the patient's condition, the more complex the problems the nurse must identify and address. Not surprisingly, it takes years

of education and experience to prepare someone who not only can assess, design, deliver and evaluate patient care, but does so in partnership with patients and their families—no mean task when you are dealing with a culturally-diverse population in varying stages of physical and mental illness, at differing educational and socioeconomic levels and in one stage or another of crisis.

2. Indeed, nurses can and do teach a patient how to care for himself or, if that is not possible, nurses will teach one or more family members how to care for their loved one. However, neither patient nor family members need learn any more. If, for example, a nurse is teaching a woman how to care for her diabetic husband, she need only teach her about her husband's condition—not his roommate's, not the man's in the next room, not the woman's across the hall. A patient or family member learns to care for one person—and one with whom they are intimately acquainted, I might add. They need observe only one person for his idiosyncratic reaction to drugs, possible interactions among drugs, response to treatment and the like.

3. By this point it should be abundantly clear that although nurses can teach a patient or family how to handle an isolated situation, it does not necessarily follow that an aide, multi-skilled worker or unlicensed assistive person can be taught to do the same things for many patients in an institutional setting. The level of illness is significantly higher than that generally found in the home and the complexity of care is generally far greater. Moreover, healthcare personnel are far less intimately acquainted with patients and their customary reactions than are family members. Moreover, they also are held to a far higher standard of care than are family members.

In short, although there is a place for the nursing assistant, it isn't at the bedside. It's at the nurse's side. Cross-training can increase the versatility and productivity of the aide, but it cannot replace the registered nurse's years of education and experience. Cross-training unlicensed assistive personnel and appropriately partnering them with RNs, however, can increase the nurse's productivity and expand the availability of nursing care, a crucial accommodation to a *universal access* world—whether or not it will reduce an institution's payroll.

Demonstrating the worth of an RN

Despite the integrated nature of health service outcomes, it may be possible to disaggregate nursing's particular *inputs*. Not only do nurses have considerable amounts of reliable data on nursing activities and work design, they also have developed a growing body of objective data on the behavioral components of service productivity. Efforts to develop a minimum data set for nursing are proceeding, as is the development of a nursing management minimum data set. Successful efforts to develop consistent language (nursing diagnosis) and classification categories have enabled economic analyses and comparison to a limited, but growing degree. Nonetheless, the problems of disaggregating specifically nursing care outcomes from health service outcomes are considerable. However, the data, taken and analyzed collectively, seem to point out measurable, identifiable outcomes of distinctly nursing interventions, none of which necessarily contradicts any of the various speculations of nursing's theorists. To wit, for purposes of economic analysis, the outcomes of nursing practice can be described as the promotion, enhancement or restoration of persons to their optimal state of functional competence. Nursing service, then, consists of nurse-patient interaction that stems from assessment of the patient's needs and levels of functioning and which is designed to optimize the patient's adaptability by integrating the efforts of patients, families, and the patient care team in such manner as to modify and/or reinforce behaviors, modify and/or reinforce various elements in the patient's environment, and provide biological care and maintenance. Nurses' claim against outcome lies chiefly in their continual presence at the interface between patient and service delivery—i.e., where the service interchange occurs. Therefore, the crucial attribute of *dependability* is measured by patients' access to professional nurses (as demonstrated by skill mix and staffing ratios) and through them, to the whole array of healthcare services and technologies. Of what use is a Swan-Ganz catheter if there is no one there to interpret it? Of what use is a pro-time, if there is no one there to translate it in terms of heparin delivery? Of what use is a medical regimen if there is no one to implement it? Of what use are diagnostic tests if the patient has not been properly "prepped" for them? At what risk are services delivered if no one has recorded their delivery? Dependability also is measured by nursing audits, nosocomial infection rates, accidents, errors, falls and the like.

To a lesser extent, the *durability* of nursing services could be measured in terms of patient's self-care abilities and deficits, recidivism rates, and discharges to home. Thus, patient teaching, discharge planning, appropriate referral for case management, reasons for readmission within specified time ranges, etc. become economic measures of the outcomes of nurses' activities.

Moreover, nursing critical paths (care maps) are the economic equivalent of small batches of products with special attributes. Individualizing them at the point-of-service tailor-makes them to specifications. For those five percent of patients whose complex needs, if inefficiently addressed, consume prodigious resources, clinically competent nurse case managers have proven to be extraordinarily effective at decreasing the cost of their care by improving the quality of their care. Combining nursing critical paths with professional nurse case management services offers an almost unbeatable—and wonderfully humane—economic package. And we even have the data to prove it.

The success of national and state health reform may well depend on the appropriate use of the advanced practice nurse. However, successful restructuring in hospitals rests primarily on the appropriate use of the registered nurse.

A number of experiments in health service delivery will be tried, but the only really successful ones will be those in which nurses remain at the heart of patient care delivery.

May 1994

Chapter 2

PROFESSIONAL ETHICS: MAINTAINING VALUES IN A PRAGMATIC WORLD

A COMPELLING STATE INTEREST?

Her hands are so contracted that her fingernails cut into her wrists. Six years ago she lost consciousness following an automobile accident. She's never regained it. Four weeks after the accident, surgeons implanted a gastrostomy tube in her stomach, and she's still here—sort of. She's in a persistent vegetative state, and she's only 31 years old. Her family wants the feeding tube removed. Missouri's Supreme Court said no. The United States Supreme Court agreed last August to hear the appeal. In any real sense, she's no longer a person. Her name is Nancy Beth Cruzan and she's become a Symbol—for both the Right to Die and the Right to Life groups. Ms. Cruzan is in limbo in more ways than one. May God have mercy on her.

A diminished quality...

The Supreme Court of Missouri, in explaining its verdict, said that "A diminished quality of life does not support a decision to cause death." Who could disagree...but, there must be *some* distinction between "a diminished quality" and the total devastation of a person: that massive and permanent brain damage unfortunately accompanied by a functioning brain stem. There also seems to me to be a very important difference between causing death by lethal injection or even withholding foods and removing artificial means of feeding. When these conditions co-exist—i.e., a persistent vegetative state *and* artificial interventions—it doesn't seem reasonable to say that removing the artificial interventions *causes* death. An automobile accident was the cause of death. I suspect what's happened to Ms. Cruzan since then is an appalling misuse of technology occasioned by the almost paranoid fear of liability that characterizes U.S. healthcare today. We demand legal protection, so we go to the courts. And the courts produce public records. And patients become symbols for competing public interest groups. And both human compassion and common sense are lost in a welter of political rhetoric and publicity.

Preventing mayhem

In its decision regarding the Cruzan case, the Missouri Supreme Court asserted that the state's interest does not lie in assessing the quality of life, but rather in maintaining life. Try as I might, I cannot see what compelling state interest is served by forcing Ms. Cruzan, her family, others *like* her, and their families to suffer a "fate worse than death." The state's compelling interest lies in preventing citizenry from murdering one another. Or even in preventing citizens from shirking their responsibilities to their kith and kin. The state's interest does not lie in forcing unfortunate families into despair or in wasting its limited health resources because professionals and courts beg the questions.

Hard questions

In all fairness, the questions aren't easy ones.

• *Does withdrawal of artificial nutritional life support constitute killing?* Complex questions cannot be answered simplistically—and this question is far more complex than it looks. There is a tendency to consider the withdrawal of artificial nutritional life support under general rubric of withdrawal of medical life support measures. It is one thing to decide not to resuscitate a terminally ill patient; it is quite another to starve a person to death whether or not he has some hope of survival. Among those aspects unique to (or exacerbated by) questions of continued nutritional life support are:

1. Possible violations of basic subsistence rights protected by both moral and legal sanctions. Subsistence rights are founded in fundamental and universal human needs. Among such needs is the need for adequate nourishment. In short, while everyone does not need resuscitation or a ventilator or an artificial kidney, every human being needs nourishment.

2. While maintaining adequate nutrition is an appropriate part of any medical regimen, adequate nourishment itself is not solely within the medical prerogative. Although the use of ventilators, drugs, defibrillators and the like is initiated and discontinued by medical prescription, nourishment is not.

3. Withholding or withdrawing medical life support measures usually is justified on the basis of futility or humanitarian concern. It is extremely difficult to argue that feeding is futile or that starvation is a humanitarian undertaking.

Surely, to deprive a person of ordinary sustenance is to kill. Thus, we have a duty to feed. However, as the means of providing sustenance have become more sophisticated, what is included in this duty has become less clear. While few among us would consider bottle feeding an infant or spoon feeding a debilitated adult to be moral options, each is an artificial means of feeding. A premature infant may have too little strength to suck and thus need a special nipple for his bottle. A debilitated adult may need his food mashed. Are such minor adjustments in the feeding process optional? From these, it is a short step to the use of tube feedings for premature infants who have no sucking reflex or for adults too debilitated to swallow. Is tube feeding a medical option or a moral imperative? If digestion is impaired, permanently or temporarily, hyperalimentation is the most effective means of feeding. Is hyperalimentation morally and legally required?

> **It is extremely difficult to argue that feeding is futile or that starvation is a humanitarian undertaking.**

Here, at least, some broad though clear distinctions are possible. When feeding could be accomplished by mouth (e.g., bottle feedings with or without a special nipple, spoon feeding whether or not the food is mashed), to deliberately withhold or withdraw it constitutes killing. Neither the technology nor the financial and human cost is excessive. However, the use of tube feedings, gastrostomies, parenteral and enteral nutrition provides limited options. What constitutes these limits—the scope of morally and legally acceptable decisions, the distinction between killing and allowing to die—is not always clear. The Supreme Court could help by setting the legal guidelines. Or it could beg the question by deciding on Ms. Cruzan's case alone.

> **If people have any rights at all, they have a right to life—even in the face of imminent death.**

• *Does imminence of death alone justify deliberate starvation of a person who could eat normally?* If people have any rights at all, they have a right to life—even in the face of imminent death. If the right to life means anything at all, it means one has a right not to be killed. Providing normal sustenance to a dying patient imposes no excessive risk or loss to anyone. However, the adequacy of the nutrition may vary depending upon the person's condition, prognosis and volition. Terminal patients may be fed on demand (and then only those foods they particularly desire) and dying infants may be fed on demand only enough to keep them comfortable. In the face of inevitable death from some other source, nourishment is used to provide comfort—and any means of feeding that produce more discomfort than comfort can be eliminated. In some cases, patients can clearly tell us what they want, in other cases we must rely on our own judgments, in all cases the goal is patient comfort.

• *Does normal feeding in and of itself constitute an inhumane prolongation of inevitable death?* Every person must die; some of us sooner than others, some of us with more pain than others, some of us more "naturally" than others. But how a person dies is not without moral significance. Surely, if a person can eat and drink, he has a right—an ordinary human right—to that sustenance. To attempt to end suffering by inducing death through starvation and dehydration is morally repugnant.

• *Do some artificial nutritional life support measures constitute an inhumane prolongation of inevitable death in certain circumstances?* In situations in which death is inevitable and the conditions of living intolerable (involve extensive technological isolation from human touch, futile pain and pointless extensions of dying), highly sophisticated means of feeding are not in a patient's best interests and may be withheld or withdrawn.

• Once started, it is psychologically difficult to justify withdrawal of artificial means of nutritional life support when death follows its removal. In situations in which sentient life is a reasonable expectation, nutritional life support measures (including hyperalimentation) generally should be continued unless a rational adult patient refuses them. When permanent unconsciousness can reliably be predicted—as is the situation in the Cruzan case—artificial nutritional life support may be terminated.

The President's Commission for the Study of Ethical Problems in Medicine (1983) had this to say: "*Most patients with permanent unconsciousness cannot be sustained for long without an array of increasingly artificial feeding interventions—nasogastric tubes, gastrostomy tubes, or intravenous nutrition. Since permanently unconscious patients will never be aware of nutrition, the only benefit to the patient of providing such burdensome interventions is sustaining the body for a remote possibility of recovery. The sensitivities of the family and of care giving professionals ought to determine whether such interventions are made.... When all remedial attempts have failed to bring the patient out of chronic coma, but where the patient is able to spontaneously maintain respiration and circulation, it would seem to be a matter between physician and family as to whether or not other, more mundane, care would continue...if the family feels the emotional or financial drain too great and the physicians in attendance indicate no reasonable possibility of any recovery, then it can be anticipated that the courts, when presented with petitions for appointment of a conservator with power to refuse consent to further treatment of any kind, including I.V. drip...can be expected to grant such requests.*"

Clearly, the Missouri Supreme Court did not. Perhaps the U.S. Supreme Court will.

The courts aren't the best place

By and large, courts are not necessarily the best places to make decisions of this kind. As the President's Commission pointed out: "judicial review is costly in terms of time and expense; it can disrupt the care of the patient; it can create unnecessary strain between professionals and surrogate decision makers; and it exposes private matters to public scrutiny and to the glare of public media. Occasionally, it may be wiser to request judicial review, but in most instances internal review by an appropriate committee is far more desirable. Institutions are urged to develop clear, explicit and publicly available policies regarding how and by whom decisions are to be made for patients who lack adequate decision making capacity." Moreover, institutions are urged to exercise their responsibility to protect patients' well-being by establishing ethics committees.

Obviously, humane and compassionate care for patients, or for families, can no more be guaranteed by a committee than they can by a court. Such private matters—family matters—do not lend themselves to public disposition. Compassion resides in human beings and is demonstrated in human relationships. Courts and committees strive to ensure appropriate procedure—and are designed to contain abuses—but, let the people most intimately involved make their own decisions within these limits. In this middle ground lies the path of salvation. Welcome home, Ms. Cruzan.

October 1989

A GIFT OF MANY PARTS

Abe and Mary Ayala didn't want any more children. They were so sure of this decision that Abe had a vasectomy. Two years ago their 17-year-old daughter, Anissa, developed leukemia. No suitable bone marrow donor could be found. Abe had his vasectomy reversed and Mary was impregnated. Prenatal diagnosis confirmed that the baby's bone marrow was HLA-compatible with Anissa's. Baby Marissa Ayala was born last April to serve as a bone marrow donor for her older sister. Abe and Mary said they had to do everything they could to save Anissa. They have. Most people only donate tissue or blood or an organ: they contributed a baby.

When Baby Marissa is six months old (the delay is planned so the baby will grow and produce enough bone marrow to give Anissa a fighting chance), Dr. Patricia Konrad will transplant about 12 ounces of her bone marrow to her sister. A successful transplant offers Anissa a 70 to 80 percent chance of a cure.

Anxiety makes poor decisions. Fear often makes brutal ones.

But what happens if she's not cured? What if she needs more of Marissa's bone marrow next year? Or in five years? What if some crisis precipitates the need for the transplant before Marissa reaches six months? Surely no one would deny Anissa access to the bone marrow of a child who was conceived to produce it for her?

The Ayalas assured the world that, while they'd never have had another child if Anissa didn't need a donor, they would not have aborted Marissa if she wasn't a match (unlike the parents of a boy afflicted with Wiskott-Aldrich syndrome who intended to abort any HLA-incompatible fetuses who would have been unsuitable donors). As the mother said, "If it's not a match, we'll love our baby just the same."

Perhaps they would have done so. Surely they would have tried very hard to do so. Nonetheless, the child would have failed to fulfill the only purpose for which she was conceived. She still may: although preliminary tests look positive, no one will know for sure until the cells are matched on the day of surgery. Even if the surgery is a success, the transplant may still fail. Studies have been done of siblings who donated their kidneys. When the transplants failed, they carried a burden of guilt. No matter that it's irrational. How much more so for Marissa? It is possible to have a child for one reason, and love it for another, but how does one explain "I had you to create parts for your sister?"

The right to one's body...

Under our laws, a person has a right to bodily integrity, i.e., no one can invade the body or take parts of it away. Rights, however, are optional for right holders, therefore the person has the option of setting aside the right for something he values more highly. Thus, a person may donate his blood or bone marrow or kidneys. What makes the act right is the *person's* consent to it.

Ordinarily, when any intervention, medical or surgical, is proposed for a minor child parental permission is a precondition. If research involves minor children, parental permission is a prerequisite—and then, *of course*, the research *must* be therapeutic, i.e., it must offer some hope of benefit to the child. Moreover, the Health Research Extension Act of 1985 prohibits research on nonviable, living fetuses *ex utero* unless the research will enhance their well-being or probability of survival or unless the research poses *no* added risk of suffering, injury or death to the fetuses.

A parent's consent...

Parental consent for non-therapeutic, not to say downright deleterious and painful, interventions in a child's life are a necessary *but not always sufficient* precondition for surgery. For example, at one time, in most if not all jurisdictions, judicial review was required before a minor could donate an organ to a sibling. While ordinarily it is presumed that parents will act as advocates for each one of their children, there was concern that the parents' anxiety and fear of the loss of one would influence their judgments about the other, healthy sibling. Anxiety makes poor decisions. Fear often makes brutal ones. At the very least, fearful people make poor advocates.

While it is true that donating bone marrow is relatively low risk, it's *not* riskless. No one could claim that taking 12 ounces of bone marrow out of a six-month-old baby will enhance the baby's health or improve its chances for survival. Surely no one with a speck of integrity could claim the procedure is pain free or that six-month-old babies don't feel pain.

Would you subject your own six-month-old child to such a procedure to benefit someone else's child? Would you have your six-month-old baby donate 12 ounces of bone marrow to yourself? Your father? Your spouse?

To donate one's own tissues or organs is an act of love. To contribute someone else's is another matter altogether. The Ayalas want to do everything they can to help Anissa. But make no mistake about it: it is Marissa whose bone marrow is being given away. Can the Ayalas really be her advocates when they conceived her to donate her tissue?

Of the ends and the means...

No one can doubt the parent's good intentions: they want to save their daughter's life. To do so, they are willing to rear—and love—another child, a child whom they hope can help the other. These are good things and the Ayalas undoubtedly are good people caught in a horrible nightmare. But the issues are very grave indeed.

• Our new technologies offer new possibilities, new hopes and horrific new choices. No human being should be created to be used as a source of spare parts for someone else...even though our technology makes it possible. A human being has a purpose, a destiny, a goal, an existence of his/her own. However many times this ideal has been trampled into the ground; to compromise human rights endangers everyone. A human being is not simply something to be used.

• The very foundations of parental consent are seriously suspect when a child is conceived to be a donor. It could be the newest form of child abuse—and we're by no means ready to cope with it.

> **No human being should be created to be used as a source of spare parts for someone else.**

• What makes this problem all the more urgent is the increasing capability to use our young to cure ourselves. And the young are powerless. And when their parents love the ones their bone marrow or islet cells or brain cells could benefit, what then? Recently, my son was talking about "cannibalizing" an old car to fix a newer one. Shall we "cannibalize" new generations to repair the old? All the while telling ourselves that we older ones have greater value because we have a higher level of self-consciousness?

What of the woman who sought to be impregnated with her father's sperm and abort at seven months to donate her fetus' brain cells to treat her father's Parkinson's disease? What of the woman who sought to create a child to provide her husband with a kidney?

• What makes the problem hit home right now is this: reportedly, about 30 percent of bone marrow donors are under one year of age. Their parents didn't go public: the Ayalas did. We were all skating on ethical thin ice. And we did not know it—or, more likely, chose to ignore it. We can't anymore. Now we must face the issues. And we must thank the Ayalas, and pray for them. And pray for us all.

June 1990

MOVING TOWARD UNITY...

There comes a time in life when one feels an overwhelming desire to communicate belief to others. I have felt such a desire on three occasions.

    • The first was when, as a young nurse, I became convinced that nurses had a great destiny—that nurses would someday bring health and hope into the ghettos of our cities and the hills of our countryside. I believed that nurses could provide care for most people under most circumstances if only our organizations and systems could be changed to allow nurses to practice effectively. I devoted my life to nurses and nursing, to surveying everything from our education to our care modalities, to "preaching", wherever people would listen, that nursing's only limits are self-chosen.

    • The second time was when I saw nurses and physicians, my colleagues, substituting a reductive knowledge of health and disease for direct knowledge of life and suffering. I believed that the tendency to view the body as a machine ("which part is not working?") and life as a scientific phenomenon inadvertently lead us to *cause* suffering. So irreversibly comatose patients are dialyzed, irreversibly dying patients are resuscitated. For 15 years, at home and abroad, I spoke, wrote and argued for a renaissance of professional ethics.

    • The third time is at this moment—in 1991. We are now facing problems intensified by years of frustration. We are in the grip of a scientific—even mechanistic—reductionism, caught in a vicious cycle where tests are done to protect personnel from litigation rather than to diagnose patients, where technology is used to perfuse tissues rather than save lives, and decisions are made on the basis of an organ's function rather than a man's life. All of which inevitably leads to horrendous costs (in human *and* material terms) which, in turn, drive us to consider rationing "care" or even adopting mercy killing as a "solution" for those who are denied care.

    Much of this is due to a paradigm that has run its course. The scientific paradigm—the basic idea that science offered an objective and rational way to look at reality that did not depend on our religion or beliefs—offered promise and hope for the future. It offered us control of life—similar to control of machines. It swept away the old medieval system which had prevailed for hundreds of years. The medieval world, the "Dark Ages," of feudal politics, mythic traditions and religious miracles paled under the glaring light of science...or so we thought.

While to some extent this was true, it wasn't the whole truth. In all honesty, the medieval system didn't work anymore. It didn't work economically. It didn't work intellectually, and it didn't accommodate the new world that was emerging.

Today, the scientific paradigm is hundreds of years old, and like the medieval system before it, it is beginning not to fit the world anymore. The paradigm finally has become so powerful that even the simplest human being can see its limits. Largely through science, we have learned to "control" nature—to prolong life, to harness the atom, to make poisons. But it cannot tell us when to stop prolonging life. Or not to build a nuclear reactor. Or not to use pesticides. And our world is being polluted in fundamental ways—air, water and land. And medicine—whose warrant is to relieve sickness and suffering—is subverted to increasingly esoteric matters. We do multiple organ transplants while thousands are denied basic services.

In an interview over Radio Brazzaville in 1953, Albert Schweitzer stated "...Certain truths originate in feeling, others in the mind. Those truths that we derive from our emotions are of a moral kind—compassion, kindness, forgiveness, love for our neighbor..." As an interesting aside, recent research indicates that selfless love, a caring for others without worrying about benefits to oneself, is related to good health. James McKay, a Harvard graduate student working under the aegis of psychologist David C. McClelland, notes that selfless love is reflected not just by thoughts of doing things for others without consideration of personal benefit but also such things as a sense of humor and a lack of cynicism.

In a series of studies, McKay found that people whose fantasies showed a tendency toward selfless love reported having fewer infectious diseases. Moreover, an assay of their T-cells showed a pattern reflecting resistance to viruses.

These results support the findings of a study by Dr. McClelland (*The Journal of Personality*, May 1991) in which the immune function was assessed in people before and after they watched a film about Mother Teresa and her work with the poor of Calcutta. In most people who watched the film, there was a significant, though temporary, rise in a measure of defense against upper respiratory infections. And when people were asked to spend an hour recalling times they had loved or been loved, the immune measures stayed at the higher level the entire time. It seems that emotion (love?) has a place in our healing.

To return to Dr. Schweitzer, "When man sets himself as a unity of reason and emotion, to meditating and to reasoning, emotion and reason are in accord." This unity is integral to any understanding of life or of suffering. In a recent essay (*Hasting Center Reports*, May-June 1991), Eric Cassell notes that "...suffering [is] the distress brought about by the actual or perceived impending threat to the integrity or continued existence of the *whole person*...by whole person I do not mean solely the whole biological organism..."

Our knowledge of human beings, their health and disease must be colored by our understanding of their hopes and dreams.

Today, we are moving from a mechanistic view of mankind and the world to a biological view. But even that is insufficient. The scientific paradigm which has arisen in the last three centuries must embrace the scholastic paradigm which dominated the three preceding ones to create a *Generative View* for the 3rd millennium. In this view, reason and emotion, past and future are held in harmony as human beings make decisions. And the cutting edge of the scientific paradigm finally will be directed by compassion.

August 1991

...GENTLY INTO THE NIGHT

"Yea, though I walk through the valley of the shadow of death, I shall fear no evil..." (Psalm 23).

In the wake of the U.S. Supreme Court's Cruzan decision which sharply limits family decisions about life-sustaining treatments for incompetent patients, Congress enacted the Patient Self-Determination Act.

This Act requires hospitals, nursing homes, and hospices to advise patients, *on admission*, of their right to accept or refuse medical treatment. Providers also must tell patients that they can execute an advance directive in case they no longer are able to express their wishes. Moreover, home health agencies and managed care organizations are required to provide this information to each of their clients upon enrollment.

All institutional providers are required:

• to document whether patients have signed advance directives

• to develop and enforce policies which adhere to *state statutes* about the execution and implementation of advance directives

• to educate their staffs, patients, and communities about advance directives.

Compliance with the Act is a condition of Medicare and Medicaid reimbursement.

The Department of Health and Human Services has installed a nationwide toll-free number purportedly to answer questions from patients and providers. However, repeated calls resulted in cut-offs, hang-ups...and no information.

Good intentions aside...

While the framers of the Act clearly intended to benefit patients, family members, and even providers, the Act may end up having little impact. For example, the Act requires that patients be informed of their rights under *state* laws which sometimes end up being *less than* their rights under the U.S. Constitution. Only 43 states have Living Will Statutes and many of them limit applicability only to terminal patients who meet certain conditions. For example, some states require that a patient be declared terminal by two physicians. Moreover, the physicians must use the criteria set forth in the statute to determine whether or not a patient is terminal—and the criteria require that a patient be practically moribund! In addition, the patient has to survive two more weeks in this moribund condition and reexecute his Living Will before it takes effect. Most states also exclude feeding tubes from among those items which may be removed at the request of patients or families—a situation which is likely to result in more Nancy Cruzans.

Among the most conservative of a conservative breed, hospital attorneys are likely to advise their clients that an advance directive which goes beyond state law should not be followed with "advance" court permission.

Moreover, a hospital admitting department is, at best, a poor place to discuss delicate subjects. In fact, "discussion" is unusual—the provision of multiple documents for patients or family members to sign in record time is common. If questions are asked they rarely are answered. If the forms aren't signed, admission and treatment will be delayed at best and denied at worst. Nonetheless, the implementation of the Patient Self-Determination Act is likely to be reduced to yet another form to be signed in the admitting department.

Two recent studies (Cotler, et al., 1991, and Tarnowski, et al., 1990) indicate that consent forms typically require reading skills at the advanced college level; most forms have an average readability comparable to that of the *New England Journal of Medicine*. Therefore, it's no surprise that providing patients/families with written consent forms rarely increases their understanding of the procedure in question. Given the complexities of state laws and the paranoia of many hospital attorneys, I suspect that "written information" on advance directives will be as readable as Kant's *Critique of Pure Reason*. Only God can understand that treatise, and even that may be open to debate.

To make it work

To fulfill the *spirit* of the Act—to make it work the way it was intended to work—state and federal officials must insist that materials provided state clearly that patients:

1. have a Constitutional right to accept or decline life-sustaining treatment and that state courts almost certainly will permit patients to exercise this right through an advance directive.

2. can execute advance directives whether or not their state has passed "Living Will" legislation.

3. don't have to use official forms, hire an attorney, or limit their directives to only those situations covered by their state laws.

Providers should urge patients to talk to their physicians about advance directives. Nurses should be prepared to discuss advance directives with every patient upon admission—as a routine part of their admitting assessment.

In the end, I still don't think laws, however well-intentioned, automatically ensure humane treatment or sane decisions. I strongly urge patients, providers, nurses and physicians—everyone—to encourage people to appoint decision-makers who will have durable power of attorney. Urge the passage of enabling legislation at state levels. And, by all that's holy, appoint one for yourself. Someone who knows you. Someone you can trust. And someone who won't be either emotionally overwhelmed by—or likely to benefit from—your death. Do it now. In today's technology-driven, liability-riddled hospital, it may be your only real chance "to go softly into the night...."

November 1991

PRIVACY: BELONGING TO ONE'S SELF

The most intensely personal aspects of every person's life are lived in silence—protected and screened from the outside world—experienced in one's secluded inner core. In a very real sense, these private experiences constitute what it is that makes one belong to oneself. It is for this reason that people jealously guard their privacy.

The philosopher, Albert Camus, put it this way: "...a man remains forever unknown to us and...there is in him something irreducible that escapes us." Although healthy people are willing to disclose a part of themselves to acquaintances, friends and loved ones, there remains an inner core that almost never is shared. Ordinarily, the amount and type of information disclosed correlate closely with the intimacy of the relationship. In certain trying circumstances, urgent circumstances, or desperate circumstances, intimate disclosures may be made to virtual strangers. One such circumstance often is the therapeutic encounter.

The use of the word "encounter" is deliberate, for it means merely "to meet face to face." Whether or not the encounter leads to the development of a relationship (i.e., a connection) is another matter.

A therapeutic relationship

People come to health professionals when they need help. Some are angry, some confused, some shattered, all are vulnerable. Their need forces them to ask for help. The health professional's response to this need determines whether a truly helping relationship will be established. To help someone, a professional must know that person—what he thinks, feels, hopes and fears. To risk disclosure of the private self, a client must believe the professional can help, will not reject, and will protect his or her confidences. Under any other circumstances, intimate self-disclosure to anyone other than a loved one would be overwhelmingly intrusive. In essence, a therapeutic relationship is one in which an artificial intimacy is imposed by the need for help.

The word privacy has as its root the Latin word *privatus* which literally means "belongs to oneself." To reveal at least a part of the protected, secluded self—a far more significant exposure than that of a body part—the client must trust the professional. If a person does not or cannot trust the professional (or sometimes even if he does), he or she may deliberately or inadvertently digress, conceal crucial material, or dwell on matters that are only minimally relevant to the existing problem.

Regardless of the fact that trust is essential to professional practice, it is not something freely given or automatically owed to one by virtue of professional status; it must be earned. To gain trust—and to be worthy of it—professionals must keep in mind what their commitments both promise and imply. The very nature of a therapeutic relationship infers confidentiality, whether or not the professional explicitly promises to maintain silence. In fact, the inferred promise of confidentiality actually enables the relationship to develop.

> **The more information one person has about another, the more control he exercises over him.**

The philosopher J. A. Austin made the now-famous distinction between two different kinds of statements: descriptive and performative. While the descriptive statements merely describe, transmit, or reveal reality, performative statements actually alter reality by introducing an ingredient that would not be there apart from the statement. The promise of confidentiality, whether implicit or explicit, is the ingredient that alters reality enough to enable the artificial intimacy of the therapeutic relationship. Precisely because the promise alters reality, to make or to break it is a serious thing to do.

The elements of privacy

At its simplest, privacy is defined as freedom from the unwarranted intrusions of others. Although the boundaries and limits of privacy vary somewhat from culture to culture, unwarranted intrusions on privacy generally include: 1) the physical presence of unwanted persons, particularly when one is engaged in an intensely personal activity; 2) unwanted observations of or by persons; 3) dispersion of private information about persons; 4) the spread of inaccurate or misleading information about persons; and 5) encroachment on personal decisions made in one's own sphere.

According to Charles Fried, the real issue is one of control: Privacy is not simply an absence of information about us in the minds of others, rather it is the control we have over information about ourselves. The more information one person has about another, the more control he exercises over him. The more vital or intimate the information, the greater the power of the one and the vulnerability of the other. In some cases, the information possessed by the professional is so fraught with peril for the patient (e.g., an AIDS patient), that disclosure can mean disgrace, abandonment... the life of a pariah. In such situations exquisite care must be taken to protect the patient while at the same time treating the patient and fulfilling reporting requirements. No mean task!

Disclosure of information for professional or learning purposes

All codes of professional ethics, frequently buttressed by statutory requirements, impose special obligations on professionals to protect patients' or clients' privacy. Patients' or clients' private lives or problems may not be exposed to public scrutiny or censure—and the "Public" means anyone not involved directly in the case of an individual. In recent years, however, some States have passed laws which forbid the release of information about one disease (AIDS) to anyone other than the patient, thus, no one but the physician may know the patient's diagnosis unless the patient expressly permits such disclosure. Ordinarily, the informed consent of a patient or client is sufficient to authorize the release of information. Not only the disclosure of information about clients, but also the setting and manner of disclosure are of concern. Even when valid

consent is obtained, special precautions should be taken to minimize the intrusion. Patients or clients are private persons, not public properties. No doubt, some sharing of private information about
patients, and even videotaping or filming may help students and
practicing professionals to learn. However, appropriate precautions
must be taken to protect clients' personal privacy. On no account
should a client be displayed like a guinea pig, as was the custom in
the 19th century. (A moving example of this practice is depicted
graphically in the play and movie, *The Elephant Man*.)

Disclosure of information to protect others

There are exceptions to the professional's duty to maintain confidentiality; for example, the legal requirement that gunshot wounds
and venereal diseases be reported to the appropriate authorities.
However, public reporting should not be confused with public
exposure. All efforts still must be made to protect the individual's
privacy.

Not surprisingly, the courts have frequently held that disclosure is warranted if there is good reason to believe the client's
actions or intended actions may bring harm to himself or others.
However, inquiries from employers, social agencies, schools, and
so forth often are excessive when judged against the need.
Especially when they touch on past mental illness or on certain
diagnostic information, such inquiries can be acutely embarrassing
and sometimes unfairly damaging to the person involved. No outside body typically stands between the inquiring agency and the
subject to determine what information really is required. The professional's discretion and fidelity to the promise of confidentiality
have traditionally been the client's major source of protection.
Recently, professionals' concerns about the possibility of civil
recovery for patients harmed by a breach of confidentiality have
added impetus to efforts to restrict access to information about
patients.

The current conflict about confidentiality for AIDS patients
adds another dimension to an already complex matter. Technically,

the reporting of information as required by law does not violate the patient's right to privacy. Nor should the sharing of diagnostic information about a patient among those who actually are involved in his care violate a patient's right to privacy. However, real concerns—unfortunately validated by experience—about the integrity of professionals have led to a flurry of legal activity as patients seek to protect themselves, and lawmakers seek to protect the public. Neither seems to be succeeding too well at the moment.

A civil right to privacy

Under United States law, a civil right to privacy that encompasses the making of certain decisions (*Roe vs. Wade*, 1973), the use of one's name or picture (Prosser, 1971), and the use and dispersion of information collected in certain private record systems (e.g., patients' records) is developing. Particularly since the 1973 United States Supreme Court decision in *Roe* vs. *Wade*, in which the Court carved out a qualified constitutional right to privacy, healthcare institutions and professionals have exhibited greater concern for patient/client privacy to protect themselves from legal redress.

Professionals, when they conduct in-house patient care conferences for those not involved directly in a patient's care, when they prepare lectures for public or professional audiences, when they write for publication, or when they conduct research, must be especially sensitive to issues of client privacy. Moreover, release of private information to other people, schools, social agencies, or employers should be undertaken carefully and only with the informed consent of the client. Even when engaged in fulfilling legal requirements for reporting information about patients, all efforts should be made to prevent public disclosure. Our professional commitments and legal duties require nothing less. The information we possess belongs to someone else, it has been given to us in trust, and we have promised to maintain it in confidence.

April 1992

Of Commissions, Omissions and Just Plain Missions

Mark Twain was fond of telling this story of a small town's pastor trying to raise money for his church. The little church was literally falling apart in disrepair, and the pastor made an emotional appeal for help.

Great was his surprise when the most miserly of the townsmen rose and offered to start the fund with a contribution of five dollars. As he spoke, a bit of plaster fell and hit him on the head. A trifle dazed, he rose again and said, "Reckon I'd better make that fifty dollars." From the back of the hall came a pleading voice. "Hit him again, Lord!"

...of commissions

These were precisely my sentiments when the Joint Commission on Accreditation of Healthcare Organizations (JCAHO) announced that it was adding four more seats to its 24 member board—three are designated as public member seats, and the fourth is an at-large nursing seat. Two seats, including the nursing seat, will be filled in 1993; the other two will be filled in 1994. "The new nursing seat acknowledges the vital role of the nursing profession in addressing quality of care issues," said Dennis S. O'Leary, M.D., JCAHO President.

> **"The new nursing seat acknowledges the vital role of the nursing profession in addressing quality of care issues."**

"Hurrah, hallelujah and 'hit him again, Lord,'" say I!

Now it only remains for the American Nurses Association to become one of the Joint Commission's corporate members. The Joint Commission's corporate members are the American Medical Association, the American Hospital Association, the American

College of Surgeons, and the American Dental Association. In 1990, the Board of Commissioners of the JCAHO was changed to include two public members; now another three have been added. One more "hit" (adding the ANA) and the JCAHO will fulfill its goal which, according to Dr. O'Leary, is to create "a community of patient interests around our Board table."

Of omissions...

The Joint Commission released *Hospital Accreditation Statistics* for 1987-1989 which presents standards compliance data for the 5,326 hospitals that had full accreditation surveys in 1987, 1988 and 1989. The book focuses on the 12 performance areas for which 30 percent or more hospitals received contingencies, i.e., were cited for less than satisfactory compliance. A full 63 percent of hospitals received contingencies for safety management, 56 percent for quality assurance activities, 50 percent for monitoring of surgery and 43 percent for drug usage.

According to Dr. O'Leary, these *very high* contingency rates are not cause for immediate alarm. Maybe not, but they sure ought to be a cause of immediate concern and swift correction...especially those contingencies which deal with "monitoring surgery" and "drug usage."

To quote Charlie Brown, "Good Grief!"

Of missions...

With fifty-six percent of hospitals receiving "contingencies" for *quality assurance* (QA), is it any wonder that the *quality improvement* (QI) movement is overtaking hospitals? Continuous quality improvement (CQI) consists of a set of tools and skills including interfunctional coordination, zero defects, costs of quality, comparisons against others' performance, and statistical quality control. More than any of these, however, CQI requires not only a different attitude, but an entirely different philosophy.

Lately I've been thinking that our parents and teachers inadvertently sent American kids the wrong message when we were growing up. When it comes to "goodness," it seems to me, we were all brought up on litanies of "don'ts," instead of "do's." The more I think about that, the more I believe that we got the wrong message from that kind of preaching, teaching and discipline. It led us to believe that, if we don't do anything "wrong," we are doing all we ought to do. We are being "good." So, "good" was "keeping out of trouble." "Good" was not "sticking our necks out." "Good" was doing nothing.

"Good" or "goodness" does not consist in the suppression of evil (wrong, bad, etc). "Good" isn't merely "blameless," it is "virtuous." "Good" isn't simply decorous, it is "altruistic." "Good" consists of doing something that is desirable or beneficial.

On nurturing goodness

In a book (*Rescuers*, NY: Holmes & Meier Co., 1992), authors Gay Block and Malka Drucker chronicle the stories of 105 remarkable people from 10 different countries. They were "ordinary" people—some rich, some poor, some educated, others barely literate, some were believers and some were atheists—who saw horrors of Nazi terrorism and did something about it. They hid Jews and other refugees from the Nazis: they risked their lives out of compassion "...we did what any human being would have done," said Johtze Vos, 82, who saved a dozen Jews in Laren, Holland.

By insisting on their "ordinariness," the rescuers underscore the idea that altruism is accessible to all. According to author Drucker, "You don't have to be a better person than you already are in order to do good." To single them out as "paragons" lets the rest of humanity off the hook.

When Nechama Tec, author of *When Light Pierced the Darkness: Christian Rescue of Jews in Nazi-Occupied Poland*, did her research, she found that rescuers were hard to categorize. "But on closer examination you see a series of interrelated characteristics." The rescuers tended to be individualistic, i.e., less likely to follow group norms. And most of them had a history of doing good deeds—taking in stray cats, visiting shut-ins, helping poor students. "They just got into the habit of doing good," she says. "If they hadn't perceived that pattern as natural, they might have been paralyzed into inaction."

Nurses are people who have chosen "doing good" as their profession.

The rescuers also tended to be tolerant: they found bigotry to be small-minded. And, while few of them planned to be "rescuers," all of them saw Jews and Gypsies (and the others who were persecuted) as human beings.

Moreover, the majority of the rescuers believe that goodness can be cultivated, that it can grow and can spread. Helena Melnyczuk, who with her father and brother sheltered Jews in their home just across the street from a Ukranian police station, says "Good is like flowers growing in certain soil. It is natural in every human being, but it must be nurtured and cultivated."

Apparently one becomes good by doing good. It is well to remember that nurses are people who have chosen "doing good" as their profession. Anyone who is a nurse could earn as good or better a living doing something else. Yet nurses have chosen to do more than sell a skilled service for personal gain. One spreads good by modelling "goodness." The same is true of excellence in practice and in patient care.

You nurture goodness in yourself each time you choose to do good and, at the same time, you inspire others to do the same. Goodness is catching. Excellence is catching. That's the heart of the mission.

May 1992

PROFESSIONALISM: FOR SALE TO THE HIGHEST BIDDER?

Dr. Arnold Relman, former editor-in-chief of the *New England Journal of Medicine*, fears that his profession has lost its ethical ways. In the *Atlantic Monthly* (March 1992), Relman argues that doctors are not, and should not be, businessmen, and yet contemporary pressures are forcing more and more of them to act like businessmen. For patients and for society as a whole, the consequences are deleterious. I urge all of you to read his article "What Market Values are Doing to Medicine." Ponder its message and ask yourself, "What are market values doing to me—and to healthcare services: hospitals, clinics and the professionals who work within them?" Are health services *public services* or are the knowledge and skills health professionals acquire actually private commodities to be peddled in the open market place?

What is a profession?
The question of whether or not healthcare is a public service necessarily involves what it means to be a professional. The word profession has as its root the Latin word, *profitere*, literally "to declare publicly." The ancients applied it to certain occupations because the practitioners of those occupations stated publicly, i.e., promised publicly, to meet certain standards and to dedicate themselves to serve the people of their communities.

The philosopher J. L. Austin developed the now famous distinction between two different kinds of statements: descriptive and performative. Descriptive statements transmit information. For example, "The tree outside my window is 40 feet high" or "You have cancer of the lung." Performative statements alter reality by introducing a new ingredient—something that would not be there *apart from the declaration.* For example, "I will help you." Precisely, because a promise is a link between what is and what will be, to make or to break a promise is a very serious thing to do.

If we intend to understand the nature of professional commitment, we must examine the performative statements of their professions. To what have professionals committed themselves? What promises are entailed in the practice of their professions?

Briefly, all health professionals have promised to help those who are ill to regain their health, those who are healthy to maintain their health, those who cannot be cured to optimize their potentials and those who are dying to live as fully as possible until their deaths. Making such serious promises entails an *honest* commitment to their fulfillment.

Honesty as fidelity

By and large, the question of honesty among health professionals has been limited to discussions of whether to tell the patient the truth (or part of it) or, more saliently, *who* should tell the patient the truth. However, the performative statements of a professional expand the demands of honesty in a professional's life. The moral for the professional is not simply a matter of telling the truth, but also of *being true* to the promises of the profession. That is, honesty among professionals not only entails truthfulness, but also fidelity.

For professionals to practice effectively, they must have the public's trust. There is no such thing as a right to be trusted; it is a privilege that one merits. To bestow trust upon a profession, the public must experience performative truth. To trust a professional, a patient or client must believe (1) that this individual has the knowledge necessary to help him, and (2) that this person will act in his best interests. The first involves knowledge: what special expertise does the professional have that enables him or her to address a specific problem? The second involves fidelity: the promises the *profession* and the *professional* both make and imply— *and whether those promises are kept.* That is, does the individual patient experience performative truth?

Because the degree of trust the public bestows upon a profession rests squarely on the shoulders of individual practitioners, the consequences of the presence or absence of fidelity in their individual members are enormous.

Unfortunately, professions develop unevenly because the professionals who comprise them are in diverse states of awareness, intellectual attainment and commitment. The dominant social values of their times also affect them. Our society has just emerged from three decades of technological advance—and at least two decades of unabashed social acceptance of ostentation and greed. The people who are professionals cannot help but be influenced by this experience. What is a wonder is that traditional professional values survived at all!

> **Health professionals have been remarkably lax in developing adequate systems to care for long-term, chronic and disabled individuals.**

Certainly, practitioners' perceptions of their roles and their character traits affect the problems they see, the personal presence they bring to them, the manner in which they address them, and the reservoir of personal resources they can call upon to serve another day. At the same time, their moral commitments (or lack of them), as repeated in thousands of their colleagues, create or destroy a profession.

Ethics in healthcare delivery

In general, ethical reflection in the context of healthcare has focused on the discrete quandaries which individual practitioners face. Obviously, professionals want to resolve the moral problems of everyday practice. Less obviously, quandary ethics tend to ignore problems of professional discipline because it concentrates on particular problems of usually anonymous practitioners. While professionals concentrate comfortably on procedural questions of appropriate decision-making, larger questions about the social and economic structures within which the profession operates are left to others—political scientists, social engineers, health planners, economists and administrators.

Concentrating only on specific, individual problems has led to neglecting the demands of social justice. Nonetheless, professional practice requires knowledge and skill essential to the public welfare; therefore, it is a public good. Public goods nourish and preserve public welfare. A just public policy requires the delivery of such essential public goods to the *whole* community. In return, society bestows upon those who serve the public good power, status and privileges to the extent that they help meet the public's needs.

The demands of justice

Clearly, no one professional or profession at large can meet all the needs of the public. In fact, a profession cannot even fulfill its own circumscribed mission without widespread communal support and assistance.

However, the principles of distributive justice impose at least four obligations on professionals: (1) to do what they reasonably can do to meet the need for their services; (2) to do what they know how to do competently whether or not the patient can pay for their services; (3) to help design methods for dealing with the health as well as the illness needs of the populace, and (4) to testify on the basis of expert knowledge to the community about the injustice of a social system that fails to meet the fundamental health needs of its citizenry.

These obligations obtain not only because of one's role as a professional but also because a professional is strategically positioned to observe the injustices that result from the inequitable distribution of health resources. With this knowledge comes both the power and the responsibility to speak out.

Health professionals have been remarkably lax in developing adequate systems to care for long-term, chronic and disabled individuals—largely because little money has been allocated to their care. While society has fostered elaborate specialization in acute medicine, it has devoted a woefully small amount of its resources to the healthcare needs of this largest segment of the population. Action goes where the money goes?

If medicine and nursing are to continue to be justifiable and viable professions, they must regain and nurture a sense of commitment—of vocation—in their members. The knowledge they possess and the skills they exercise are more a public trust than a private asset to be prized and sold on the open market. The contemporary climate which encourages physicians and even nurses to center on their personal economic status places their professions in extraordinarily vulnerable positions because money is far too narcissistic a focus for a profession; i.e., an occupation which claims to merit both the public trust and social privilege.

Opportunities for financial gain and personal advancement within a profession flourish only in the context of the valuable services that the profession provides to the public: the utility and the advancement of a profession depend on individual members who have some sense of professional identity, commitment, and responsibility. When each practitioner thinks of himself or herself as an entrepreneur—alone, unencumbered by a public and professional trust—the professions are wounded, perhaps mortally.

By virtue of their traditions and their social contract, medicine and nursing can ill afford to deny their public function, the interdependence of their practitioners, or their inherently altruistic goals. To the extent to which market values are embraced by the professions, the moral fiber of the professional will be weakened and the activities of the profession itself will be reduced to commercial transactions. The dictum *caveat emptor* (let the buyer beware) certainly is not an appropriate motto for any profession. If the virtues of public service—and the presence or absence of them in each profession—do not prevail, the vast resources of the professions will be for sale to the highest bidder.

June 1992

MIRROR, MIRROR ON THE WALL

In *You Don't Have To Be in Who's Who to Know What's What*, Sam Levenson twists a line from a legend into a joke. "Mirror, mirror on the wall, who is the fairest here of all?"

And the mirror replied:

"You are, you are! But don't go by me. I'm cracked."

Joe or not, the facts which mirror the performance of hospitals have been organized and catalogued in book form by the editors of *Consumers' CHECKBOOK* magazine. Entitled the *Consumers' Guide to Hospitals*, it covers such topics as "How to choose a hospital," "Death rates at 6,000 hospitals," "Best hospitals for specific types of cases," "How to get the best care wherever you go," and "Cutting your hospital costs."

Based almost entirely on Medicare data, the image it presents may be "cracked," but it's the best thing—at any rate, the only thing—available to consumers written in language that the average college graduate can understand. Not only does this *Consumers' Guide* present data, it also gives advice. And it is instructive for us to review the advice it gives.

In the chapter on "How to Get Good Care...," the editors offer these kinds of advice.

• **Monitor your own care:** "...learn as much about your care as possible...during treatment keep notes on the results of tests, and changes or effects of medication or diet...write down questions...and record the answers."

• **Be yourself:** "...try to personalize your day or your surroundings...do all you can for yourself...be sure to express your appreciation for the good care you received...learn your nurses' names, and call them by name."

• **Be aware of your rights:** "...a few guidelines will help you judge the quality of care you are receiving:

"1. Nurses should observe you every few hours if you are not seriously ill—every few minutes if you are.

"2. They should answer your calls at once.

"3. They should spend time with you to ask about any changes in your condition, any pain, any new complaints.

"4. They should call your doctor if an unexpected change occurs.

"5. There should be some continuity of the nursing staff—not a constant daily turnover of new faces."

At the outset, the *Guide* advises consumers that "...hospitals remain today, as they always have been, dangerous places. The fact is dramatically illustrated by malpractice case records which reveal operations done on the wrong patient or the wrong organ, heart attacks caused by feeding the wrong solution into an IV hookup, infections passed among patients...inaccurate lab or x-ray results, administration of unprescribed medications and slow response to emergencies.

"Although all hospitals are dangerous, some are certainly better for your health than others...Quality questions have taken on a special urgency since 1983 when hospitals first began to be...paid a fixed amount per patient...As a result, a hospital can achieve surplus income by cutting the costs of serving each patient..."

Whatever you think of the *Consumers' Guide to Hospitals*, one thing is sure: you can expect to see more and more comparative information on hospitals in newspapers, magazines and hospitals' own advertisements.

Patient satisfaction

What *do* patients want? According to the *Consumers' Guide* they want:
- no complications;
- improvement in their conditions or ability to function;
- improvement in, or at least maintenance of their morale; and
- a pleasant (under the circumstances), comfortable stay.

Thus, it should be no surprise to anyone that when Press, Ganey Associates prepared *The Satisfaction Report*, two of the top scoring items contributing to patient satisfaction were 1. the friendliness of the nurses and 2. the technical skill of the nurses.

Larger hospitals, urban hospitals and teaching hospitals achieved lower scores on every question. On the whole, Press, Ganey reports, "Religious ownership...appears to make no significant difference in overall patient satisfaction. While mission statements are given much attention at the corporate, strategic level...mission does not appear to make much difference at the "ground" level...Hospital organizational culture appears to have a life of its own."

> **Time was when a hospital was a place to die.**

Corporate development

Eric Reidenbach (University of South Mississippi) and Donald Robin (Louisiana Tech) have developed a five-stage model of corporate moral development. "All stages are not necessarily reached, progression is by no means linear, and one can certainly slip from one stage back to an earlier one" reports the *Journal of Business Ethics* (November-December, 1989, pp. 13-14). "The Stages:

"I. **The Amoral Corporation**—pursues winning at any cost and views employees merely as economic units of production...may violate societal values and rules...

"II. **The Legalistic Corporation**—is concerned with the letter of the law and adopts codes of conduct that read like products of legal departments (which they are)...

"III. **The Responsive Corporation**—is interested in being a responsible corporate citizen, but primarily because it is expedient, not because it's right; has codes of conduct that begin to look more like codes of ethics...an understanding that ethical decisions can be in the company's long-term economic interest even if they involve an immediate financial loss...

"IV. **The Emergent Ethical Corporation**—recognizes the existence of a social contract between the business and society, and seeks to instill that attitude throughout...balances ethical concerns and profitability...

"V. **The Ethical Corporation**—balances profits and ethics so completely that employees are rewarded for walking away from a compromising action; includes ethical issues in training; has mentors to give moral guidance to new employees...*starts out* with a founding moral stance that permeates the culture..."

The researchers could find *no* examples of the Stage V Ethical Corporation....

Perhaps they could not because they did not look in the right places.

Hospitals as ethical corporations

Among the items I treasure in that select collection of readings and clippings to which I return periodically, I have an old yellowing copy of the *Menninger Quarterly* dated Summer, 1954. It contains an article by that extraordinary human being, psychiatrist Karl Menninger, written on the occasion of the opening of a new building. He said:

"Time was when a hospital was a place to die. It was not a place of mercy and of healing, but one of endurance, charity, and pity. But the meaning of the modern hospital is quite different. It is no longer an asylum, no longer a pest house, no longer a hotel on the way to God. It is a beacon, a lighthouse—and for all its scenes of suffering, it is a place of joy. It is a place in which people come, not to die, but to cease dying—a place in which to get well. Temporary refuge it may be, and in another sense from the original, truly a 'hotel of God'—and way station, not on the way to death, but on the way to life."

Whenever I hear criticism of our healthcare institutions, I return to this statement, a founding "moral stance" that, with all their flaws and warts, permeates hospitals' corporate cultures. That is, unless they've lost their stance to unbridled competition and a bottom-line mentality.

But the founding vision, the moral stance, is kept alive through the policies the corporation adopts and through the behavior its leaders model. To return to Dr. Menninger's quote:

"Even as we sit and look at these walls, and touch them with our hands, walk upon the solid floors, and admire the physical beauty, we know that all this is not the hospital. Like the corrupting mortal flesh in which eternal spirits are housed, a hospital building is only a shell in which the meaning of a hospital can be realized. So what is the meaning of a hospital? The meaning of this hospital is embodied in the fabric of the personalities, the human beings, who work together in it."

In the end, the corporate culture is founded in the professional person—in the character of the individual and in the kind of relationships that constitute his or her life.

While an uninterrupted siege of disapproval is bound to be irksome, the feeling of being under scrutiny is not altogether unhealthy. It can provide the impetus for self-examination and growth. The historian Arnold Toynbee saw the process of progress, or at least change, as emanating from what he called "challenge and response." Today, we call it CQI.

The publication of books like the *Consumers' Guide to Hospitals* emphasizes the scrutiny we are under. The Press, Ganey *Satisfaction Report* underscores patient expectations, namely that they really do expect hospitals to deliver human and humane services. And Reidenbach and Robin's model of Corporate Moral Development offers one more tool to help us examine and measure, not just what we do, but who we are. "Mirror, mirror on the wall..."

September 1992

THOUGHTFULNESS: SOMETHING WE HATE, NO DOUBT

I live in Cincinnati, Ohio. That may not mean much to you, but an awfully lot has been happening in this city lately—the kinds of things that represent in microcosm some of the problems that beset our society. Cincinnati was voted the #1 most livable city in the United States in 1993. I believe it. I love this place, but...Christmas was marred by the Ku Klux Klan which erected its sacrilegious symbol of hate on our famous Fountain Square. Moreover, Cincinnatians passed an anti-gay rights amendment in 1993, even though our newly elected mayor offered to act as spokesperson for the Gay community.

Of course, our problems cannot compare to New York's: so far no one has entered a commuter train and shot people to death because he hates the color of their skin. Maybe that's only because we don't have a commuter train.

We versus they...

Reading about Bosnia, Northern Ireland, the Mideast, fundamentalism, backlash, skinheads—and the Long Island commuter train—it seems that the world (and with it our communities and workplaces) is falling deeper into bigotry. The "we vs. they" or "us vs. them" mentality makes thinking simple for the bigot.

We consists of the group with whom the speaker identifies. They can refer to people of a different race, sex, religion, skin color, language, political party or sexual preference from the speaker's. They also can easily be expanded to include those of more or less education, wealth, power and so forth. The operative word here is different. They differ from us in significant ways.

We are inherently physically, mentally and morally superior to them. We, of course, are all that is good, noble, thrifty and, above all, deserving. They, on the other hand, are all that is greedy, lazy, dishonest and, above all, *undeserving*. If *they* happen to be success-ful (especially if they are more successful than *we*), envy turns "superiority" into hate and malevolence leads to violence. Violence in word and deed is justified because, as all right-thinking people know, *they* have to be kept in *their* place (or, in some cases, elimi-nated altogether) because *their* existence threatens the right order of things.

Bigotry's baneful presence...

Bigotry is nothing new: history amply demonstrates its baneful presence. In fact, it is so historical that it's practically Neanderthal, and at least as brutish. Not all violence, however, is physical. Lots of it is attitudinal and, quite frequently, verbal. *We* are smug; sure that what we are, do or believe is superior. *We* **matter** more than *they* do; therefore, *we* deserve more. Rather than hurl rocks or burn crosses, we build walls (or ceilings?) of exclusion (so much more civilized!). *They* are ignorant: unaware of their own "inferiority" and try to penetrate the barrier—which reminds me of a wonder-ful, even if apocryphal, story:

Innocently unaware of the prejudices held against him, Jack Johnson, the great black heavyweight champion, applied for membership in an "exclusive" church. The pastor, fully aware of the prejudices of his "flock," tried as tactfully as he could to put him off with one flimsy excuse after another. Jack, becoming aware that he was not wanted, finally told the pastor that he would pray about it and then get back to him in a few days. The problem was that this was the only church of his denomination convenient to him in the community in which he now resided.

Several days later he returned.

"Well," asked the minister, "did the Lord send you a message?"

"Yes sir," was the answer, "the Lord told me that it was no use. The Lord God said, "Why, Jack, I've been trying to get in that Church myself for over 10 years, and I still can't make it!"

A few cases in point...

Exclusion, prejudice, pain. Over the years every one of us has paid a devastating price either because we were its victims—or because we were its perpetrators: narrow-mindedness allows us to become not only more shallow, but infinitely less vital, and certainly less humane, human beings. There is no surer way of achieving perspective on this issue than by experiencing it.

• When I was teaching at a local university, one of my students asked me to give her some work to make up for the time she would miss while she celebrated Rosh Hashana with her family. I gave her an assignment and thought nothing more about it until she came back to me for help. The director of the nursing program threatened to dismiss her from the nursing school if she took this "unauthorized" time off. Despite my interventions and, eventually, the Rabbi's attempts to influence her, the director would not budge. The student took the time off, and the director expelled her from the school. Miriam was devastated, but undaunted. I helped her get a job as a nursing assistant in a Roman Catholic extended care facility (they were *delighted* to find someone who didn't mind working Christmas!) and led a faculty campaign to get her reinstated. She was reinstated and went on to graduate with high honors...and the profession of nursing gained a brilliant and compassionate member. But the student lost a year of her life.

> **Narrow-mindedness allows us to become not only more shallow, but infinitely less vital, and certainly less humane, human beings.**

• An American acquaintance told of her experience while traveling by air in Japan. She speaks Japanese, and was startled to overhear a conversation between the flight attendant and the Japanese passenger who was seated beside her. The flight attendant was apologizing to the man for the indignity he suffered by being placed next to an Anglo. Fortunately, the passenger was gracious. When, later in the flight, my acquaintance responded to the flight attendant's query in fluent Japanese, the woman had the grace to look chagrined.

• While traveling on Delta Airlines, I was stranded in Atlanta. After waiting in line for some time to get a standby seat on the next flight to my destination, I was shocked to be informed by an admittedly harried ticket agent that they would be accommodating the business men first. He kindly, if condescendingly, informed me that business men travel frequently. Apparently he assumed that because I was a female, I traveled infrequently, and then only for pleasure. Possibly because I have travelled over two million miles on Delta **on business**, I was literally rendered speechless (a rare circumstance indeed!). Later, after checking his computer, he apologized: although none of the seats opened up, if one had I would have been given it because I had flown more miles than *anyone else on that flight*.

• At the International Conference of Nurses' meeting in Tel Aviv, I fell into conversation with a Nigerian nurse, an earnest young woman of boundless curiosity. During the course of a lengthy discussion, she asked many, many questions about nursing in the U.S., and expressed wonder whenever the talk turned to social values. At one point, she asked me what I thought was one of the most intractable problems I had dealt with in my practice as a nurse. Without hesitation, I said "Child abuse." She asked why I did not just tell the parents to stop hurting their child and, if that failed, why didn't I go to the head man (mayor?) and tell him that I was displeased. This is what she would do—and had done on those rare occasions in which she had encountered child abuse. I tried to explain our beliefs and laws, and why such an approach would not work here. After listening to me for some time, she said, "That is the saddest thing I have ever heard. In my country, all of the people in a town are responsible for all the children, and they

> **The only way to begin to overcome bigotry is to focus on our similarities.**

know it. In your country, it seems that parents own their children, and what they do to them is no one else's business."

Legally that isn't exactly accurate, but attitudinally she was right on the mark. My unquestioned assumption that the U.S.A. is a "first world" country because, with all their flaws, our ways are better than those of "third world" countries suffered a massive jolt.

Obviously, these are not earth-shaking events, but they represent bigotry in minor key. Bosnia represents bigotry in major key. Minor key bigotry also is hazardous: it deprives people of opportunities and sows seeds of bitterness that ultimately poison society. In the workplace, it certainly will be counterproductive and probably disruptive. At the *very* least it deprives organizations of that success which comes from putting the right person in the right place to do the best job.

Focus on the universals...

As each year melts into the next, business comes closer to realizing the multi-ethnic workforce of the future. For the most part, the literature approaches cultural diversity by emphasizing understanding of and respect for differences in values, behaviors, and beliefs. This is great. It really is. But it **still** focuses on *differences*...And focusing on differences, even though well-intentioned, can lead to a condescension which is itself a form of prejudice. In his autobiography, Frederick Douglas, a famous 19th century black author and civil rights advocate, described his visit with President Abraham Lincoln: "Lincoln is the only white man I ever spent an hour with who did not remind me that I am a Negro." His point is well taken. Lincoln related to him on a more fundamental level, a human level: quite literally *man to man*.

The only way to begin to overcome bigotry is to focus on our similarities. Human beings really **are** more alike than they are different. No matter how different people may seem, they all need food, shelter, and meaningful work. They want their children to have a decent start in life, and they seek success. Most understand the need for education. Most want acceptance. All need respect. I need, you need, *we* need, *they* need, we all need self-respect which enables us to be mutually respectful.

My daughter Rose once told me that she stopped seeing a man because he was rude to waiters, and I understood perfectly. Someone who is rude to waiters or sales clerks or business "subordinates" undoubtedly will be found wanting on all major issues. People live their values everyday, reflexively, in a hundred tiny ways. In the end, you are your values and value choices.

Any business which allows, or, God forbid, *fosters* bias through its policies and the behavior of its leaders ultimately will be found wanting in all major ways. Businesses, corporations, live their values everyday, reflexively, in the policies they proclaim, the procedures they implement, and in the decisions of their leaders—in thousands of ways. In the end, the conduct of their business (and its success) reflects the values and value choices it embodies.

Over the years, I have learned that it is naive to estimate the contents of people's hearts on their ethnic, religious or political affiliations—though listening to any of Rush Limbaugh's programs always gives me renewed pause—but the principle remains valid. We all have our own perspectives and beliefs, and I guess we think they are right or we would not hold them. However, when they harden into bigotry and envy turns them into hatred, *we* are the ones who become less than human.

In the final analysis, it is a matter of tolerance, based on respect, and manifested through consideration. On the face of it, showing consideration for others shouldn't be a terribly difficult proposition. It really doesn't take any more energy to be thoughtful than to be thoughtless, but somehow it seems that few of us are able to manage it. Something we hate, no doubt!

February 1994

QUALITY, THE OLD FASHIONED WAY

I hate to be called an old fogey, although this title places me in imminent danger of being so labeled, **but** I'm having a problem with the notion that competition always and inevitably improves quality. To be sure, a social system founded on individual achievement and self gratification has its pluses: some people are, indeed, driven to great accomplishments. Take Tonya Harding, for example, a world-class athlete whose competitive spirit drove her to outstanding achievements. Nonetheless, she stands accused of plotting to disable her rival, Nancy Kerrigan.

Whether or not she is eventually convicted, one is led to ask, "Why would anyone so talented, who worked so hard, who had achieved so much, *why* would a person like *her* do such a thing?"

The obvious answer is *to be absolutely sure of winning.* Incapacitating a competitor is justified (so the thinking goes) because a competitor is an *enemy.* There is no such thing as a contest in which one demonstrates superior ability. There is only war. And there is no such thing as losing fair and square. Enemies rob you of what is rightfully yours, and so they become someone whose loss is something to revel in.

The Tonya Harding situation is no different from football players who **try** to injure an opponent or fans who **cheer** when a player on an opposing team is hurt. My third grade teacher, Mrs. Bloomers (that really was her name) had a word for it: **Envy.**

According to Mrs. Bloomers, "envy is a coal that comes hissing hot from hell." She'd then quote from the Gideon Bible each of us kept in our desks (this was before the Supreme Court decision outlawing them): "envy and wrath shorten life."

Corroding the human system

Nothing so corrodes the soul as an advanced case of envy: an emotion by no means confined to sports! Envy (one of the seven deadly sins, Mrs. Bloomers would have reminded us) is largely a matter of self-contempt—or, at the very least, a profound (though unac-knowledged) dissatisfaction with who one is. Not that those driven by envy are likely to perceive this: they are truly persuaded that if they had a little more luck or opportunity or chutzpah, what the other person has would be theirs.

Last Spring, I was having lunch with a friend at the AONE convention. She had just changed jobs and, with salary, bonuses and perks, was now making $20,000 a year more than in her pre-vious position. She was on top of the world—until I told her about someone we'll call "Mary," at which news she choked on her pizza. Rumor has it that Mary is making $800,000 a year as a consultant. "All that money for *that!*" she finally managed to say. "Why doesn't that kind of money ever come my way?"

"Probably because you wouldn't be willing to sell nursing down the river," said I, feeling not at all guilty about having taken the wind out of her sails.

"Yes," she said, "the world isn't a fair place."

Notice how we turned "Mary's" good fortune into something we could look down on. The notion that Mary may be more talent-ed or harder working is just too painful to acknowledge.

Unfortunately, healthcare in general—and nursing along with it—has recently become *competitive* and thus particularly suscepti-ble to the tribulations of galloping envy. Virtually everyone in healthcare is jealous of someone else. Administrators of one hospi-tal are jealous of another's marketshare. One health plan is after the other one's customers. Dr. Hardy (of *General Hospital* fame) undoubtedly is jealous of Dr. Casey and so on.

Not that people in healthcare circles are any more subject to envy than anyone else: assistant professors are jealous of tenured professors, lawyers are jealous of other lawyers who have larger practices, business men are jealous of other business men who have bigger offices, even mothers are jealous of other mothers whose daughters may be chosen to be cheerleaders. A good case could be made that the entire economy is fueled by envy.

And, in the end, unbridled envy is the one thing that could bring it down.

Thy neighbor's praise

Unlike anger, love, grief, guilt or even shame, there is nothing therapeutic about envy. Envy consumes the envier, robbing him of the pleasure he might otherwise take in his own accomplishments, in what he has and does. Self-pity follows envy: poor me, I don't have what you have. And, as surely as night follows day, indignation follows self-pity: I deserve what you have. So, I take it away from you.

Even in its lesser stages, it is an ugly little scenario: envy not only elicits a slew of our baser traits—backbiting, petulance, gratuitous nastiness—but usually does so in an embarrassingly public fashion. Inevitably, we end up looking bad.

I met one hospital administrator who actually was angry because a board member from a competing hospital was honored for his humanitarian service to the poor. Another one who was livid because a competitor was cited as *best in class* by a publicly-sponsored rating agency. And a third who actually fought with his wife because she said something nice about the chair-person of another hospital's board.

Even if we manage to say a few words of praise about a competitor's success, we can't pull it off without saying something to diminish the accomplishment. It's *impossible* to envy someone with style, the emotion itself is too petty. Which, by the way, is not to say it isn't part of the human condition (remember, Mrs. Bloomers quoted *Scripture*, for crying out loud, to the effect that envy shortens life—and they only lived to be about thirty back then!).

Lest you think I am being disgustingly self-righteous about all this, I confess that I have spent a considerable amount of time gnashing my teeth over some really great articles published in other people's journals, like *JONA, AJN,* and *NAQ.* Not to mention my distressing tendency to wish I had written many of the wise and witty lines already published by others.

A common vision

Even though envy is an integral, if lamentable, part of the human character, one also must note that it thrives particularly well under certain conditions. There is comparatively little envy in situations in which people share common values, adhere to common beliefs and work together for mutual ends. Unity of purpose—for example, the way all of us pull together in an emergency—allows us, at least for that period of time, to feel utterly at one with those around us. With mutual goals and a common vision, competition is swept aside and all cooperate to the common good.

Continuous Quality Improvement (CQI) and Total Quality Management (TQM) and all the rest of our efforts *ought not to be about* **being the best**. They ought to be about **doing one's best**. Not measuring yourself against others, but measuring you against yourself. Not measuring your unit against other units, but against itself. Not trying to beat competitor hospitals at what they are doing, but about determining what your hospital (agency, health system) can do best—and then doing it for all you're worth. Values must be overhauled and ways of thinking changed.

Managing the risks of truth decay

I read somewhere—perhaps it was in Sam Levenson's book, *In One Era and Out the Other*—that we are living in an era of "truth-decay". While contemporary philosophers debate the advisability of honesty in one's personal and professional life ("How do you know if honesty is the best policy if you haven't tried some of the others?"), pop psychologists urge us to can the conscience (an anachronistic harbinger of guilt) and shed the shame which used to accompany dishonorable behavior.

A little dishonesty (lie-ability?) is not only accepted, it has added considerably to our **liability**. If dishonesty is socially acceptable and widespread, no one can believe anyone, and everyone has to check up on everyone else, including health professionals and providers. So much so that lie-ability has become really big business, adding dramatically to everybody's workload.

In healthcare, documentation requirements now account for a startling percent of the cost of care as patients and payors demand proof in writing that we did what we said we did. And institutions have had to establish whole quality assurance and risk management departments to act as a substitute conscience for caregivers who used to have one of their own.

Meanwhile, private insurers have taken to hiring their own inspectors to inspect our inspectors to make sure the charges we are charging are ones they actually owe. And then there's the government with all its rules and penalties and inspections. The GAO estimates that over one-third of the increase in health costs is associated with trying to be sure that health providers are being honest.

Of course, no one trusts the government to be honest, so we hire lawyers and other specialists to assure that we get what the government honestly owes us. Thus, we have watchers watching the watchers who are watching the watchers who are watching the caregivers who are watching the patient.

A little bit of dishonesty is very expensive.

The quality continuum

When we were nursing students (most of us, anyway, back in the "old" days when hospital schools "trained" nurses), our instructors used certain words which were intended to teach us how to be "good" nurses. They were woven into basic *nursing arts* courses, *professional adjustments*, and clinical practicum. They were our value words, our moral primer back in the days before ethics courses.

The primary words I refer to were courtesy, kindness, respect, accuracy, duty, loyalty, commitment, justice, honesty, diligence, compassion, discipline.

Let us take, for example, the age-old ethical norm (and foundation of the nurse's notes) "Honesty is not only the best policy, it's the **only** policy." Honest and timely reporting had the moral support of countless nursing instructors, head nurses and nursing supervisors. Not only did we report what happened, including (God forbid!) any errors, we also reported any "near misses." **It was expected**—and our consciences (not to mention our faculty) would have killed us if we had failed to do so.

From there we moved into *Harmer and Henderson* (our nursing Bible), learning what the nurse does for the patient (what he would do for himself unaided if he could), the importance of "aseptic" technique, our social role and proper professional deportment. We never doubted our intelligence (only the top ten percent of high school graduates were permitted to enter a nursing program) or our ability to learn quickly (we worked 40 hours a week, attended classes 20 hours and had to study and socialize in what was left).

We were indoctrinated and inspired by stories of Florence Nightingale, Clara Barton, Lillian Wald, Ann Breckinridge, and Genevieve de Galard-Terrause: those nursing **overcomers** who achieved greatness despite the odds. By the time we were ready to graduate, we had learned the words which spelled out the character of the **ideal nurse** and of us, nursing's earnest apprentices.

At commencement exercises, the class valedictorian always reviewed the "standard" professional standards our honorable faculty had inculcated in us as they led us up the rocky road of professional Achievement and Integrity, carrying the Nightingale lamp in their hands as a beacon to light our path through the darkness of illness and despair.

We were never to forget—or fail to remember—the Trust placed in us, the Lives which depended on our judgment, or the Responsibility we bore to promote our noble profession. These were the keys to success: hardly a source of envy for anyone.

It was made clear to us in a thousand ways that the moral values which sustain the profession were not to be undermined in deed or even in thought. Whether we knew it or not, we shared a common vision.

This vision, and the values which sustain it, led us to the pursuit of a "quality" healthcare system. It still does.

March 1994

A Codified, Systematized Death?

*To every thing there is a season, and a time to every purpose
under the heaven;
A time to be born and a time to die...*

Ecclesiastes 3:1-2

Last October I lost that rarest of all gifts, a true friend.

I remember the day she told me about the lump she'd found in her breast. I stood beside her when she called her family physician of more than 20 years: he couldn't "fit her in" for at least two weeks. *It was a large lump,* but she trusted him...so she waited. He referred her to a gynecologist whose secretary also could not find any time for her for several more weeks. *It was a very large lump,* but she trusted the system...so she waited. When the gynecologist referred her to a surgeon, his staff could not possibly give her an appointment for another two weeks. *It was a very large angry looking lump,* but she had no choice...so she waited.

Following her radical mastectomy (the tumor was virulent and rapidly growing), the surgeon informed her that he had found cancer in all but one of the lymph nodes he'd removed. He referred her to an oncologist.

Carolina did not have a strong will to live, she'd lost that years ago when she was pressured into resigning her post as a high school teacher. The Vietnam War was raging and some students refused to say the Pledge of Allegiance. She advised them to talk to their parents about loyalty and patriotism, and what should be included in a Pledge. The newspapers got a hold of it and made out that she was a subversive—and worse. She often said "they" killed her when they destroyed her reputation.

Thus, she was inclined to refuse treatment until we talked about how much chemotherapy and radiation can relieve pain, improve the quality of life...and decrease one's dependence on others. That did it (when you know someone really well, you know just where and how to turn the screws). Proper (she planned to earn her millions by writing a book entitled *Confessions of an Unrepentant Virgin*), proud, and very intellectual, she was appalled—not by death, nor even by the daunting prospect of irremediable suffering—but by the humiliation of progressive dependence on others for her personal needs. She asked me there and then not to let that happen to her. "Promise me," she said in a voice as close to pleading as she was capable of sounding.

The oncologist ordered a bone scan, and I went with her to get the results: she had multiple mets—principally in the spine. Carolina was stoic...so I cried for her that night.

For years Carolina and I had engaged in intellectual debate. She was my chief researcher and confidant. I valued her keen mind and intuitive insights. But, though she little understood it, I valued her good sense and good heart even more:

• She helped rear my children, taking them to museums and historic sites, actually believing in their desire for intellectual development despite evidence to the contrary.

• She offered her home to a Vietnamese refugee family and lived in her own basement for a year until they could get their feet on the ground.

• Later she volunteered to foster two teenagers whose mother committed suicide.

At first she responded well to the chemo and radiation therapies, but after a year's remission, she suffered her first pathological fracture. Another bone scan revealed many more sites of metastasis. She wanted to understand, so I took a picture of a skeleton and marked each site in red. It made a sobering picture. She said, "If all those bones break, I won't be able to take care of myself anymore." I said, "No, probably not."

I got every bit of information I could for her—including information on hypercalcemia: how to recognize its symptoms, how easily her oncologist could treat it, and how quickly one died if it went untreated. She said she thought it was God's way of preventing bone cancer patients from suffering too much. I did not disagree.

In many ways, Carolina learned more while she was dying than she did in her 65 years as a scholar. She learned how good people could be. She learned that there were people who loved her. She even learned that human compassion is at least as valuable as intellectual insight. She learned the joys of ordinary living: she created a garden; she

There are things far worse than dying.

enjoyed her foster grandchildren; she fussed over the plight of the various young people she'd taken under her wing. In her dying, she learned to appreciate life for its own sake.

Despite a pathological fracture of the hip (she had a hip implant done the August before she died), Carolina was independent, at least where her personal needs were concerned, until pain and drugs engulfed the last three days of her life.

Of course, at the time, it was impossible to predict that she would live only three more days (the oncologist had indicated that she had "three to six months" only two weeks before). Once, when the pain medication was cut back so she could change her will, she awoke in screaming agony. After that, she was not allowed to regain consciousness again. Incapacity and drug-induced incompetence did not creep up slowly, it leapt up quite suddenly to dominate the person who had been Carolina.

It was impossible and unseemly for so decorous and cerebral a woman to "shuffle off this mortal coil" in so mean estate. "I could not stand to have others take care of me." She'd said those words in my presence, to me. And I knew it.

There was no turning death back anymore. "Her spirit already is gone, and all that's left for her body is agony or coma," I argued with myself. No one could call this *life*, so there is no life left to take, I reasoned.

Fortunately for me, nature acted before my ruminations ended. Carolina died in her foster daughter's home in the presence of those who loved her.

Physician-assisted suicide

All of this, the entire case history, is by way of saying, "I understand and I don't know the answers and I wish I did." It is an acknowledgment that there are things far worse than dying. It also is a way of saying that the debate over mercy killing is at least as emotional as it is intellectual, at least as personal as it is political.

However, this controversy is not new: debate over the morality and legality of mercy killing goes back at least as far as Plato. The term "physician-assisted suicide" only muddies the waters. Suicide itself is not illegal. It has been *decriminalized* in most jurisdictions throughout the United States. What is not legal is for someone else to help one kill oneself—not a bad idea given the violent tendencies of the human race.

Decriminalizing suicide does not mean that citizens have a *right* to kill themselves nor does it imply that the State has any duty to aid or abet citizens who wish to kill themselves. Quite to the contrary: the State and any of its representatives, health professionals, teachers and social workers—all of us—have a duty to provide alternatives to the would-be suicide. Not a bad idea, either, given the self-destructive proclivities of human beings.

> **The debate over mercy killing is at least as emotional as it is intellectual, at least as personal as it is political.**

Moreover, data support the proposition that Americans are quite successfully committing suicide even in the face of prohibitions *against* helping them do so, and considerable efforts directed toward helping would-be suicides find alternatives. It is one of the leading causes of death in the United States, particularly among the young.

There are even more data to support the proposition that the suicide of a family member *increases the likelihood—by several fold—that other members of the same family will opt for "the final solution" to life's problems.* It is interesting to note that very few terminally-ill people commit suicide, but then no one is suggesting that physician-assisted suicide be confined to the terminally ill nor even to those suffering irremediable pain. Certainly Dr. Kevorkian has not so confined himself.

Suicide centers?

It has been proposed that once physician-assisted suicide is legalized, suicide centers could be established where those who met the criteria would be helped out of this world in a safe, comforting atmosphere by skilled, caring professionals. Of course, the criteria would have to be developed carefully, and safeguards established to prevent errors and assure accurate reporting. A whole system would have to be developed, routines established, and legal accountability assured...and hierarchies created to ensure compliance...and institutions built within which all this would occur. Probably with federal funds.

Nonetheless, it would be less costly than even hospice care, not to mention the savings associated with the use of intensive care unit beds often occupied by dying patients.

It **is** cheaper to give an overdose, no doubt about it. This is not to say that there would be no money to be made: personnel must be hired, buildings and grounds built and maintained, standards upheld, and the like. Undoubtedly, each health network will want to contract with one or more. Perhaps they will even start one of their own. Moreover, drug companies will vie with one another to produce the finest life termination drugs. Industrialists will have to develop, test and market the necessary equipment and supplies. The money is in the details, so to speak.

Put aside the various philosophic and moral arguments, and think about the **practicality** of it all. *And what do we do with those who, like Carolina, can no longer speak for themselves?* Living Wills that include proxy consent for mercy killing? Durable power of attorney which includes authority to consent to mercy killing? *And what of the severely damaged neonate?* Proxy consent for euthanasia? Limited only to those not expected to live—or shall we include, like Kevorkian has, those whom some would consider to be in for a life of suffering or mental incapacity?

And what of those who, as we struggle toward a universal access system characterized by an aging population and the probability of rationing, *are denied access?* Should they be offered the assisted-suicide option in lieu of treatment? All these questions, and many more, would have to be answered and policies developed.

It is downright impossible to take a private decision, like suicide or mercy killing, to the policy-making level—to take a private act into the public arena—without institutionalizing it. In fact, the very act of taking it to the societal level codifies it. And once codified it must be systematized to prevent abuse. And institutionalized to assure access. And routinized to assure quality.

A codified, systematized, institutionalized, routinized death. A cold, formal shove into eternity—administered by strangers.

I don't know the answers, but I'm reasonably sure that being processed to die isn't one of them.

July 1994

Chapter 3

LEADERSHIP: CREATING A VISION FOR THE FUTURE

THINGS UNATTEMPTED YET

In 1532, Machiavelli wrote: "There is nothing more difficult to take in hand, more perilous to conduct, or more uncertain in its success, than to take the lead in the introduction of a new order of things.... The innovator makes enemies of all those who prospered under the old order, and only lukewarm support is forthcoming from those who would prosper under the new...because men are generally incredulous, never really trusting new things unless they have tested them by experience."

Why the resistance

Actually, Machiavelli understated the case! Anyone who has ever tried to change anything knows that—and each probably has asked the question "Why? Why do even those who have suffered under the old ways often resist change?" I'm not sure I can answer that question, but I'll try. Social scientists repeatedly report that institutional change always intimately affects the lives of the people who are its members. Occasionally institutional changes make their lives easier. Far more often, change demands greater effort for each individual—this is particularly so in the short run and, moreover, the higher up the hierarchy one is, the greater the burden that change imposes. Many otherwise intelligent people resist change because they find comfort in the familiar. Most people also figure that what worked in the past will work now. Finally, some people fear that they will lose status if they accept an idea that somebody else originated. This last "reason" for resistance is the least logical but psychologists suggest that it may be the most common.

Building commitment

Nonetheless—and despite all of the above—coerced change rarely lasts. Successful change requires commitment, and commitment comes from only one source—people. It consists of three essential elements: 1. a strong belief in the importance of the values and goals of the change; 2. a willingness to exert considerable effort to achieve the change; and 3. a strong identification with the change. To induce commitment, one must demonstrate it. Anything you do to strengthen identification with the change, strengthens the ties. Failing to explain the reasons for changes, taking cheap shots at administrators, and criticizing the institution undermines commitment.

To nourish commitment, one must provide reassurance. To reassure employees you must enunciate *clear* goals—short and long term. Tell people, *clearly*, what is expected of them and how they will be judged. Give immediate feedback and recognition: the greatest reassurance employees can receive is to be informed that they are meeting or exceeding expectations and that those in authority know it. To *reinforce* commitment, build mutual trust. Trust consists of 1. consistency; 2. caring (*response* to need)—a.k.a. *follow-through*); and 3. faith that the consistent caring of the past will continue.

The qualities of leadership

The essential qualities people look for in their leader are visibility, flexibility, authority, assistance, and feedback.

• *Visibility*—they want to know that you are around and accessible. People like to *see* their leaders. There is no substitute for presence. When you're not on the scene, people must know how to reach you and/or whom to call in an emergency.

Frequent, casual contacts are preferable, but being on hand when something goes wrong is crucial.

• *Flexibility*—people learn from leaders who can "roll with the punches," who are open to suggestions, and who keep their cool under pressure. Flexible people also delegate well and adapt to new circumstances. So do their employees.

• *Authority*—authority is not something imposed from above; it is recognition granted from below. It is the right to make decisions, give direction, accept and administer criticism. Ordinarily, authority is granted to another only when four pre-conditions are met: 1. the employee *understands* the communication; 2. he or she

believes that what is asked is consistent with the goals of the organization; 3. the communication (request, command, point of information, etc.) is compatible with his or her values and best interests; and 4. the employee is mentally and physically able to
respond appropriately.

• *Assistance*—the Roman Catholic Church's hierarchy, certainly among the largest in the world, has a motto: *servi servorum dei*—
the servant of the servants of God. Ideally, a true leader sees him-
self/herself as one who serves those who serve, create, produce.
One whose job it is to see to it that the environment and resources
necessary to do the job are in place. If you define your role as one
who sends pronouncement down, as one who criticizes, con-
demns, and bosses others, people will resist you and eventually
defeat you.

• *Feedback*—remember the law of gravity in human relations:
communication flows down far easier than it flows up. To correct
this imbalance, ask and then listen—really listen and take notes.
Always respond—and be as consistent as humanly possible. Give
people a date by which they can expect a resolution or response.
This is feedback—not the superficial pat on the back or "first name
calling" that passes for feedback in some circles today.

Technological change

All of the above is by way of introducing a new way of looking at
successful change and leadership in nursing.

Dr. Norbert Wiener of M.I.T. used the phrase "communication and control" to describe the results of developing a science
like cybernetics. Automated equipment exercises control and is
controlled by information input. Part of this process demonstrates
the principle of feedback: the machine performs, monitors its own
output, and feeds this information back to itself to adjust its own
action to new conditions. New technologies develop as the old
ones no longer yield productive results—or, at any rate, *as* productive results as are necessary to assure both a good outcome and a
healthy profit.

Ordinarily we think of technology as machines—newer, more sophisticated machines. However, new technologies also include new ways of doing things: process technologies. Machine technologies almost always give rise to process technologies. This we understand. Few of us realize that process technologies, on the other hand, also give rise to new machine technologies. And the cycles repeat and interact and accelerate change.

Nursing is a process technology—a way of doing something—and new ways of doing are continually cropping up. Moreover the machine technologies which surround us demand yet newer ways to practice. And our new ways of practice refine and create new machines and/or applications. The pace is so rapid that the half-life of knowledge is now about 2½ years.

> **A true leader sees himself/herself as one who serves those who serve, create, produce.**

To cope with these changes we need leaders who constantly reassure and reinforce what does not change—the value of the people we serve and the importance of the service we give. We need to fight constantly our own resistance to the new ways (we call it self-discipline). And we all need to evaluate the results of one change before we are plunged into yet another. To succeed—and this means to adopt those changes which best fulfill our mission—we need feedback and, above all, trust.

Nursing is a process technology, yes. But it is far more. It is a human service based upon a philosophy—a system of *beliefs*—at the root of which stands the value of the individual. If the philosophy doesn't change much, then the new technologies—both process and machine—will serve the individual. And the *profession* of nursing, no matter how much changed, will remain intact...for it will be safe for us to adopt as our motto, John Milton's phrase from *Paradise Lost*: We shall gladly explore "things unattempted yet."

July 1989

LEADERS: THE ORGANIZATION'S PACEMAKERS

Whether we want to admit it or not, values are the heart of any organization. Ordinarily, the values an organization proclaims through its philosophy and social function either attract or repel people. The organization's management system, employee policies, reward systems and decision-making tactics codify its values. Consciously or unconsciously, those who don't "fit" are selected out (by their own choice, or the organization's).

This Attraction-Selection-Attrition (ASA) Cycle automatically intensifies the degree of value consistency found in any organization. Usually, that's a good thing: the more employers, managers and employees share similar values, the less likelihood of friction, the higher the likelihood of efficiency and the greater the probability of success.

Leaders epitomize the values, define the goals which attract people, select key personnel, and develop the power, performance and reward systems. Complex interactions among the organization's environment, technology, structure and the character of its leaders determine the behavior of mature organizations.

What kind of leader are you?

By and large, people act on the basis of the meanings things have for them—meanings that are shared by the person's attitudes, assumptions, values and beliefs. Recent structural developmental research suggests that most adults inhabit one of four developmental stages: Opportunistic, Social, Goal-Oriented and Self-Defining.

• In the *Opportunistic Stage*, people tend to hold and use power unilaterally, play their cards "close to the chest," externalize blame for failure on others or situations and focus on the outside world and gaining control of it.

- People in the *Social Stage* of development tend to focus on group norms and seek approval through adherence to norms.
- *Goal Oriented* people emphasize the competent execution of rationally interrelated steps leading from strategy to implementation to expected outcome.
- The *Self-Defining Stage* of development is characterized by persons who are closely attuned to their inner feelings and to their outer environment (see Exhibit I).

EXHIBIT I

LEADERSHIP STAGES OF DEVELOPMENT

Stage	Characteristics	Behavioral Style
Opportunistic	Unilateral Instrumental Low Tolerance for Diversity or Ambiguity Concrete Conforming Action-Oriented	Self, others, & events are treated as external things to be manipulated
Social	Highly Political Cognitive Simplicity Stereotyping Low Tolerance of Ambiguity Interpersonal Focus Process-Oriented	Self, others, & events are seen as systems of behavior to be treated as technical systems to be influenced by molding one's behavior to key in on their inner workings
Self-Defining	Principled Intra-Individual Focus Autonomous Interdependent Abstract Thinker Empathetic High Tolerance for Diversity & Ambiguity Social Awareness	Self, others, & events are treated as developing systems to be influenced by creating mutually determined frameworks that permit freedom to hold different values and provide mediation of value conflicts
Goal-Oriented	Conscientious Empathetic Socially Aware Peacemakers Higher Tolerance for Diversity or Ambiguity Institution Focus Team Oriented	Self, others, & events are treated either as rational systems which respond to substantive argument and calculated action or as interactions of irreconcilable perspectives to be influenced by tolerance and discussion

In Aristotelian terms, the good leader must have *ethos*, *pathos* and *logos*. The *ethos* is his moral character, the source of his ability to persuade. The *pathos* is his ability to touch feelings, to move people emotionally. The *logos* is his ability to give solid reasons for an action, to move people intellectually.

Research indicates that most managers inhabit either the Opportunistic or the Social stage of development. The style a leader develops is largely a function of his or her stage of development. *Leadership style* describes how managers manipulate power. Basically, managers choose between collecting power by joining forces and pooling resources, or competing for access to its use by pressuring or manipulating one another (Exhibit II). *Leadership type* refers to a manager behavior profile, i.e., how he or she interacts with superiors, subordinates and with the organization (see Exhibit III).

Exhibit IV, a three-dimensional matrix, illustrates how these characteristics and traits mesh. Suppose that you like to help others achieve their goals, are really interested in the politics of your organization, and enjoy competing for rewards. On the other hand, suppose you also are willing to bend the rules to your advantage but sometimes you focus more on *how* things get done rather than on what gets done. If this description fits you, then you are *Gamesman* at the *Social Stage* of Development who exhibits a *Transactional* leadership style (see Exhibits I, II, III, and IV).

EXHIBIT II

LEADERSHIP STYLES

Style	Characteristics
Heroic	Relies on own technical skills (autocrat)
Transactional	Enables others to fulfill their goals (egalitarian)
Manager-as-Developer	Develops subordinates' abilities to share in management (educator)
Transformational	Leads others by raising their levels of consciousness about the value of outcomes and inspires them to transcend their own self-interests (charismatic)

EXHIBIT III

LEADERSHIP TYPES

Types	Characteristics
The Company Man	Goal-oriented, team player, hierarchical, methodical, gregarious Transactional style of leadership May be manager-as-developer Tends to "Headship"
The Jungle Fighter	Success-Oriented (personal & organizational), ruthless, ambitious, untrusting, C.Y.A. Autocratic, innovative, heroic style of leadership Ignores the rules
The Craftsman	Task-oriented, skillful, careful & thorough planning, precise, egalitarian Manager-as-developer style of leadership Follows the rules
The Lone Ranger	Personal achievement-oriented, entrepreneurial, innovative, autocratic Heroic style of leadership Ignores the rules, or makes them
The Gamesman	Process-oriented, political, competitive Negotiator, Bureaucratic Strictly transitional style of leadership Exploits the rules

EXHIBIT IV

LEADERSHIP CHARACTERISTICS

		Style															
		Heroic	Transactional	Developer	Transforming	Heroic	Transactional	Developer	Transforming	Heroic	Transactional	Developer	Transforming	Heroic	Transactional	Developer	Transforming
Leadership Type	The Company Man																
	Jungle Fighter																
	Craftsman																
	Lone Ranger																
	Gamesman																
		Opportunistic				Social				Goal-Oriented				Self-Defining			
		Leadership Stage of Development															

139

Profiling yourself helps you see how you fit in your present environment or points out directions for your own personal development. Profiling leaders you interact with daily not only is fun, but helps you deal with them more effectively. Profiling candidates for a leadership position can help you select the right person for the right place.

Value-based leadership

If you understand where people are coming from, you can devise tactics which tap into commonly held values. The three essential components of value-based leadership are persuasion, negotiation and compromise. To effectively practice these arts, one must first understand that what people call "truth" is filtered through different sets of ideals, values and experiences. Thus, they form different opinions about what the facts mean, what goals should be sought, and what decisions and actions are appropriate to reach the goals (see Exhibit V: The Circle of Opinion).

> **The three essential components of value-based leadership are persuasion, negotiation and compromise.**

Persuasion is the art of getting people to share a similar perception of the truth so that they can work together—with a minimum of time lost to frictional and transactional costs—to achieve the same goal. Negotiation is the art of coordinating different perceptions of the truth so people can work together efficiently to achieve a common goal. Compromise is the art of identifying and trading off non-essentials so that the integrity of each party is intact as they work together to achieve mutual goals.

Even when people agree on an ultimate goal (e.g., quality care for patients at the lowest possible costs), they may disagree about the choice of processes and techniques to be used and the spirit in which they are to be implemented. If these problems are not resolved, paralysis may set in. At best, nothing gets done and at worst, everyone fights for his personal opinions.

EXHIBIT V

CIRCLE OF OPINION

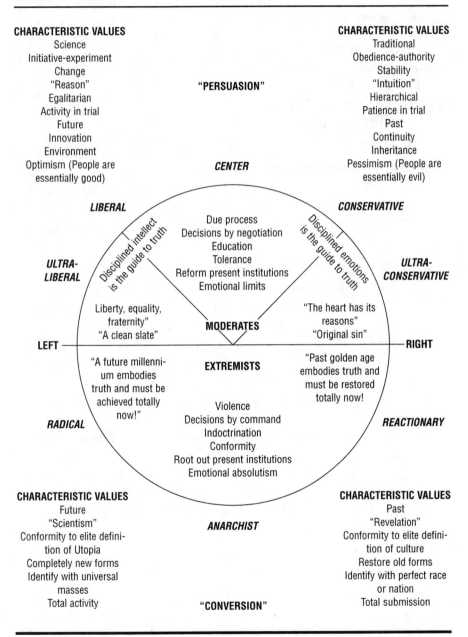

CHARACTERISTIC VALUES
Science
Initiative-experiment
Change
"Reason"
Egalitarian
Activity in trial
Future
Innovation
Environment
Optimism (People are
essentially good)

"PERSUASION"

CENTER

CHARACTERISTIC VALUES
Traditional
Obedience-authority
Stability
"Intuition"
Hierarchical
Patience in trial
Past
Continuity
Inheritance
Pessimism (People are
essentially evil)

LIBERAL

CONSERVATIVE

Disciplined intellect is the guide to truth

Disciplined emotions is the guide to truth

ULTRA-
LIBERAL

ULTRA-
CONSERVATIVE

Due process
Decisions by negotiation
Education
Tolerance
Reform present institutions
Emotional limits

Liberty, equality,
fraternity"
"A clean slate"

MODERATES

"The heart has its
reasons"
"Original sin"

LEFT

RIGHT

"A future millenni-
um embodies
truth and must be
achieved totally
now!"

EXTREMISTS

"Past golden age
embodies truth and
must be restored
totally now!

RADICAL

Violence
Decisions by command
Indoctrination
Conformity
Root out present institutions
Emotional absolutism

REACTIONARY

CHARACTERISTIC VALUES
Future
"Scientism"
Conformity to elite defini-
tion of Utopia
Completely new forms
Identify with universal
masses
Total activity

ANARCHIST

"CONVERSION"

CHARACTERISTIC VALUES
Past
"Revelation"
Conformity to elite defini-
tion of culture
Restore old forms
Identify with perfect race
or nation
Total submission

141

Because moderates agree on *overall* values and goals (and most people *are* moderates), the areas in which conflicts usually arise involve the techniques and processes chosen to accomplish the goals. The ability to persuade, negotiate or compromise, as well as the ability to convey a sense of fairness and respect, depends on the leader's ability to *understand* (not just know) the bases of both employees' and the organization's values, attitudes and opinions. To the extent to which leaders can tap into—or, at least, appeal to—employees' value systems, they compliment employees' good judgment and help *vest* the employees in the organization's success.

> **Leaders adopt strategies to reduce uncertainties, to set direction, to focus efforts and to reduce risks.**

Strategic vision

Leaders are quintessentially strategists. In fact, the root word of strategy (*strategos*) means general or leader. Just as some leaders "fit" better in certain environments, so some strategies are more suited to certain organizations. Leaders adopt strategies to reduce uncertainties, to set direction, to focus efforts and to reduce risks.

Strategy is not so much about adaptability in behavior as it is about regularity in behavior, not about discontinuity so much as consistency. Occasionally, strategies may be adopted to change the existing value structure. However, to be effective, leaders must build these strategies on a foundation of pre-existing values. Perhaps the most significant role of strategy in organizations is to resolve the big issues so that people can get on with the details of implementation. And that's how a leader keeps an organization's heart beating.

March 1991

"I KNOW YOU THINK YOU HEARD..."

I know you think you heard me, but—did **you** hear **me**? **Really?**

These days the music that fills the air (and the TV screen) is certainly full of sound and fury—not to mention smoke and strobes. While the Grateful Dead et al. drive hard to raise our consciousness, we rarely catch the words even though we can't avoid the "vibes." Somehow, despite—or maybe because of—Marshall McLuhan, the message is getting more and more lost in the medium.

There probably never was a time when people understood one another. Consider the problems which can arise when "expert healthcare" giver meets "lay" patient. In his autobiography, Frederick Loomis, MD, tells us what happened when he conscientiously examined a woman whose symptoms suggested mitral stenosis. As he searched under the patient's breast for the characteristic clinically labeled "thrill," "I closed my eyes for better concentration, and felt long and carefully for the tremor. I did not find it, and with my hand still on the woman's bare breast, lifting it upward and out of the way, I finally turned to the nurse and said, "No thrill."

"The patient's black eyes snapped open, and with venom in her voice she said, 'Well, isn't that just too bad? Perhaps it's just as well you don't get one. That isn't what I came for.'

"The nurse almost choked, and my explanation still seems a nightmare of futile words..."

> **The words we choose, as well as the words uttered in our presence, shape our reactions and the reactions of those who hear them.**

How easily we forget what powerful symbols of reality words are. The words we choose, as well as the words uttered in our presence, shape our reactions and the reactions of those who hear them. Using the wrong symbol or associating one with the wrong context can lead to baffling reactions which confound our intentions and damage our relationships.

Harvard pioneer in human relationships, Fritz Roethlisberger, noted two important ways in which words play tricks on us:

1. Because we use the same word for two or more different things, we could think we are dealing with the same thing—when a different meaning altogether was intended.

Thus, Dr. Loomis nearly got his face slapped because his patient mistook the context in which he referred to perceiving no "thrill" even though she certainly "heard" what he said.

2. Because we use different words to refer to the same thing, we think we are dealing with different things when we are actually dealing with the same thing.

Thus, I regard my stand on an issue as "firm." You regard it as "stubborn." Both of us, however, are talking about the same situation: what differs is our point of view, not our object of reference.

The great Edwardian philosopher and mathematician, Bertrand Russell, used to make fun over "scientific" pretensions to objective observation and communication. What he called "conjugating irregular verbs" showed how readily we substitute an emotional word for a rational one.

"I am firm. You are stubborn. He is a pig-headed fool."

"I am careful. You are fussy. He is a cranky, old fuss pot."

"I wear a subtle Parisian perfume. You overdo it, dear. She stinks."

In all cases, the words used to describe the same circumstances transmit entirely different messages to our emotions. And empirical research since Russell's day confirms his wry observation that what we hear is determined by the feelings the words generate rather than the objective content the words report.

Charles Goldsmith summed up international communications in a hilarious article in *The Wall Street Journal*: "Sometimes it does all get lost in translation. 'Please leave your values at the front desk,' says a sign at a Paris hotel. At a Japanese hotel, 'You are invited to take advantage of the chambermaid.' A Zurich hotel advises: 'Because of the impropriety of entertaining guests of the opposite sex in the bedroom, it is suggested that the lobby be used for this purpose.' A Swiss eatery proudly warns, 'Our wines leave you nothing to hope for...' [In Bucharest, guests are bluntly enjoined] 'The lift is being fixed for the next day. During that time we regret that you will be unbearable'... And a Rhodes tailor wants early orders for summer suits, 'because in a big rush we will execute customers in strict rotation.' ...But who needs clothing?...A laundry in Rome says 'Ladies, leave your clothes here and spend the afternoon having a good time.'..."

> **"The meanings of words are not in the words; they are in us."**

In his classic book, *Language and Thought in Action,* S.I. Hayakawa outlines five principles of good communication that are worth keeping in mind:

1. **"A map is not the territory it stands for; words are not things. A map does not show all of a territory; words never say all about anything."**

The word "lumber" is not something with which you can actually build; all it does is suggest some real objects out there with which you *could* build. Some essentials are bound to be missing; e.g., what kind of wood, how it is treated, what are its dimensions. Look behind the words, not by asking for dictionary definitions, but by concentrating on the objects or attributes the individual is trying to describe.

2. **"The meanings of words are not in the words; they are in us."**

In using words and in listening to the way others use them, always think about the people who are parties to the communication and how they perceive the words.

3. **"Contexts determine meaning."**

Suppose you stopped at a traffic light and your car won't start again. You are blocking a lane of traffic in rush hour. A stranger approaches you and says, "Got a problem, lady?" You might be tempted to retort, "No, I just love the sound of honking horns." Instead, recognizing that in this context his comment constitutes an offer of help, you answer, "Yes, my engine won't turn over, and I sure could use some help." Result: at the very least, he'll help you get your car to the side of the road—and he may even help fix your car for you.

4. "Watch out when you use generalizations."

Generalizations can serve valuable purposes: they tell you about things categories of people have in common. However, generalizations also conceal all-important ways in which people in those categories differ. All or none statements are dangerous.

When you say something, be sure you know your own purpose in speaking. Are you simply calling attention to the facts? Are you assessing blame? Do you want an explanation? Do you want someone to do something? If so, be explicit about what you want to happen. Gear your language to the person you are addressing.

When you are listening to someone, ascertain what they want—not what you want to respond. Are they venting? Do they want advice? direction? a friendly ear? What is the context? What do their words mean to them? to you?

5. Distinguish between directive and informative statements."

Are you merely passing along information, or are you trying to get someone to do something? Does the person who is speaking want suggestions from you or does he merely want someone to listen to him?

The need to talk **to** someone finds its expression in everything from friendly confidences, to the confessional, to the psychoanalyst. In fact, the need to be listened to—to be heard—is so great that people are willing to pay someone just to listen. Not long ago, an organization calling itself **The Southern Listening Bureau of Little Rock, Arkansas**, published the following advertisement:

"We offer well-trained and experienced listeners who will hear you as long as you wish to talk, and without interruptions, for a nominal fee. As our listeners listen, their faces portray interest, pity, fellow feeling, understanding; where called for, they exhibit hate, hope, despair, sorrow or joy. Lawyers, politicians, club leaders, reformers can try their speeches on us. You may talk freely about your business or domestic problems without fear of having any confidence betrayed. Just let off steam into the discreet ears of our experts and feel better."

If you are communicating well, people will tell you, "You talk my language." Or maybe they will just say "Thank you." In either case, it is a compliment of no mean order!

March 1993

WHEN PUSH COMES TO SHOVE...

Over cups of coffee, around cafeteria tables, at formal and informal meetings, nurses inevitably end up discussing the future of nursing. No one involved in healthcare today is immune from feelings of uncertainty about the future.

Bruising criticisms from all sides—payors, patients, the media, the government—lower morale while they underscore the imminence and direction of impending changes.

Pushing physicians

Nurses are gobbling with rage over the American Medical Association's latest foray onto their sacred turf. It seems the "boys" (as in "good old") released an informational report on the preparation of nurses in advanced practice. The language in the report was critical of the "highly variable" requirements for certification. This should surprise no one. For one thing, requirements for certification *are* highly variable. For another, *this is* the AMA, after all.

What is at stake is clear: primary and preventive care in America. No doubt *Nursing's Agenda for Health Reform* calls for access expansion at lower cost through use of nurses in advanced and highly specialized roles. Physicians, embattled on all sides, are left with little to hang on to other than alleging that nurses are not adequately educated for these roles. This stance is particularly ironic in view of the fact that AMA has staunchly opposed efforts to improve and/or lengthen nursing education.

The facts speak for themselves: 1) nurse anesthetists and nurse midwives have been functioning safely and cost-effectively for decades; 2) studies have demonstrated that nurse practitioners are more effective than physicians in some areas (an ANA sponsored meta-analysis of the effectiveness of NPs showed they achieved higher scores than MDs on "resolving pathological conditions and on patients' functional status as well as patient satisfaction and compliance. Their average cost per visit: $12.36 compared to $20.11 for physicians;" 3) only 1.35 percent of registered nurses—or about 27,226—are nurse practitioners so the threat to physicians is hardly overwhelming.

Nonetheless, nursing leaders know we must regularize nursing education and certification requirements and increase numbers to meet social needs. Then, nurses and physicians can work together to care for people in a reformed healthcare system. In the interim, pushing and shoving and jockeying for position continues.

Shoving hospitals

Hospital restructuring and work redesign, often euphemisms for downsizing and downgrading, raise questions about safe staffing and standards of care. After expressing concern last year that some hospitals may have falsified information, The Joint Commission (JCAHO) announced on February 11, 1993 that it will begin random, unannounced surveys nationwide starting July 1, 1993.

An ANA sponsored meta-analysis of the effectiveness of NPs showed they achieved higher scores than MDs on "resolving pathological conditions and on patients' functional status as well as patient satisfaction and compliance. Their average cost per visit: $12.36 compared to $20.11 for physicians."

The new policy provides for annually conducting such surveys for a five percent random sample of healthcare facilities which have already been accredited in the usual manner. "We expect, and clearly the public expects, healthcare organizations to be accountable. This new activity will permit us to gather accurate and objective data on accredited organizations' efforts to continuously improve their performance... Unannounced surveys...serve as a powerful mechanism for validating the self-sustaining improvement capabilities of [TQM] initiatives," said Dennis O'Leary, M.D., Joint Commission President.

All that is well and good, but then "The Joint" goes on to say: "The one-day unannounced surveys at a randomly-selected sample of accredited organizations will occur at the approximate mid-points of their three-year accreditation cycles. The content of the survey will be limited to the five performance areas, and underlying standards, that survey data for the previous year have identified as being most problematic in accredited organizations. These performance areas are specific to each of the five types of organizations that the Joint Commission accredits—hospitals and those organizations providing long-term care, mental healthcare, ambulatory care or home care services.

"The surveys will be conducted by a select cadre of surveyors in each accreditation program who will be specially trained in the use of the survey protocols. A single surveyor will conduct each survey."

All that seems just fine—sort of in line with TQM objectives and all that—but then comes the zinger: "...The survey results may lead to new Type I recommendations (areas identified as needing improvement) and may even cause a change in the organization's accreditation status, e.g., shift from Accreditation with Commendation to Accreditation, or a loss of accreditation because of an identified serious and immediate threat to patient safety.

The public have become aware of what nurses *can* do—and how cost-effectively they can do it.

"The policy will include all accreditation programs on a proportionate basis, and will cover all categories of accreditation. Moreover, the Joint Commission will continue to conduct separate 'for-cause' unannounced surveys, as appropriate. In 1992 the Joint Commission conducted 27 such 'for-cause' unannounced surveys."

"In sum," Dr. O'Leary concludes, "random unannounced surveys have considerable potential to enhance the meaning and value of accreditation."

I am reminded of that wonderful proverb that ends "...and the truth will set you free." *Indeed.*

Squeezing providers

To add to the general malaise, Mr. Clinton has proposed over $62.6 billion in Medicare and Medicaid cuts over the next five years as a "stop gap" while Congress debates health reform, et al. Fear that hospitals will shift costs to the private sector probably will result in even more scrutiny (and so forth) from private payors.

Making room for nurses

Among the few professions that can reasonably anticipate a better future is nursing. That the nursing profession has a brighter future can be surmised in part from its difficult past; in part from the enormous contributions nurses have made despite the obstacles nursing has faced; in part because—despite everything—nurses have advanced their education and created new roles; and in part because the public (and especially policy makers) have become aware of what nurses *can* do—and how cost-effectively they can do it.

There is a lot of pushing taking place nowadays. In fact, push has come to shove. For once, the nursing profession is in there with both elbows. That should boost your morale!

April 1993

IT'S NOT ENOUGH TO BE RIGHT

The profession of nursing came into being during a time of intense social change. The late 1800s and early 1900s were marked by economic instability, depression, massive immigration, demographic changes, growing labor and capital classes, violence and social disorganization—as well as exciting scientific and psychological discovery and innovation.

In that process, and as a part of it, hospitals made a transition from custodial to remedial care. Florence Nightingale played a major role in this particular social change by creating an educated and well-trained workforce that focused on the quality of hospital care and on teaching at the bedside. She believed and taught that one nursed the sick and not the sickness.

Once again an era is ending, and once again turmoil has descended on the field of health care. Indeed, it will be years before a new stability is established. Health reform, restructuring, partnering with insurance entities, managed competition and managed care, political debate, lack of access, exciting new technological breakthroughs, frightening new infectious diseases, downsizing, and the like in healthcare are occurring against a backdrop of increasing violence and social disorganization. The American Nurses Association is playing a major role in this change by helping to shape national policy and keeping the nursing community informed and active in the health reform debate. Nowhere was this clearer than at the June A.N.A. convention, keynoted by Hillary Rodham Clinton, who thanked nurses and urged them on to greater efforts this Fall.

New structures, new power

During periods of social upheaval, traditional power structures are weakened and may fail, thus new power centers can form. And new leaders emerge. For many years now, it has been clear that **the** major issues of this century cluster around the use of power—and the morality of those who exercise it.

In a century that has known the power of totalitarian governments under Fascism and Communism—under Hitler and Stalin...and Mao Tse-tung and Ho Chi Minh—only the naive believe that any system is immune from the corruption of those who wield power within it. It was none other than Reinhold Niebuhr, a leading theologian and ethical philosopher, who pointed out in the days when Hitler was triumphantly sweeping all before him that power without morality is tyranny, and that morality without power is futility. It is not enough to be right; one must be able to shape events in a world beset by conflict and change. Moral ends also require the use of power in various forms.

> **Power without morality is tyranny, and morality without power is futility.**

Even in a world as complex as ours, the decisions that are made—and their outcomes—often revolve quite simply around who possesses the power to assert social, political, professional and personal interests. Leaders emerge, hold their power and increase their power according to how they respond to the challenges of their times.

The power of an effective leader stems from several sources:

- **position power** granted by organizations, institutions or social customs.
- **personal power** derived from such qualities as character, persistence, dedication, diligence, and courage.
- **expert power** earned through education and experience.
- **democratic power** vested in the leader by the followers.

Nursing's leaders need nurses to invest them with democratic power but they lose credibility.

The people make the powerful

Unjust, or merely unrealistic, decisions often result because power has been vested in one group rather than another, because the weaker group lacks cohesion and political savvy, and because of the assertiveness of the stronger group as compared to the inarticulate, inchoate weaker group. Even those leaders who have both *expert power* and *personal power* and who have been placed in *power positions* by their organizations are likely to fail in the end without *democratic power.*

The responsible exercise of democratic power rests on the will, determination and character of the followers. Followers create their leaders and enable them to accomplish great deeds through wise selection, through their support and ability to hold steady through the storm, and through their willingness to set petty objectives aside in favor of the common good.

During the Civil War, President Lincoln frequently held public receptions in which citizens could approach him directly with their concerns. At one such "reception," a farmer from one of the border counties in Virginia told President Lincoln that Union soldiers had helped themselves not only to hay but to his horse, and he hoped the President would urge the proper officer to consider his claim immediately.

> **Even those leaders who have both *expert power* and *personal power* are likely to fail in the end without *democratic power.***

Reportedly, Mr. Lincoln said that this reminded him of an old acquaintance of his, "Jack" Chase, a lumberman on the Illinois who was sober and steady—and the best raftsman on the river. It was quite a trick to take the logs over the rapids; but he was skillful with a raft and always kept her straight in the channel. Finally a steamer was put on, and Jack was made her captain. He always used to take the wheel going through the rapids. One day when the boat was plunging and wallowing along the boiling current, and Jack's utmost vigilance was being exercised to keep her in the narrow channel, a boy pulled his coattail and demanded: "Say, Mr. Captain! Stop the boat for a minute—I've just lost my apple overboard!"

Nursing's leaders need nurses' support but they lose heart.

If we place petty concerns above the common good, we distract and disempower our leaders. The dynamics of this phenomenon was explained by Harold Lewis, dean of Hunter College School of Social Work (City University of New York) in a brilliant analysis of the power problems in health institutions. He put the questions directly: "To what extent do organizational restraints exercise power over the decisions of healthcare providers? How is decision-making to occur in today's managed care environment? Which, if any, of the professions ought to exercise power over decisions denied to others? And, if so, under what circumstances?" How ought to medicine and nursing handle the overlaps as nursing's advanced practitioners move into new areas? How ought to nurses determine which functions can safely be delegated to lesser prepared persons? What systems of responsibility and accountability need to be in place to ensure both universal access and safe care?

Questions, answers and action

These are weighty questions, but if nursing as a profession fails to ask them, or fails to demonstrate a capacity to implement the answers it offers, the body of the profession will fail to benefit from the changes currently underway in the healthcare system. Fortunately, as evidenced by nurses' growing concern with organizational structures, health networks, power and politics, nursing is beginning to ask the relevant questions. Even more fortunately, nursing has found—and documented—at least some of the answers.

To be sure, the answers are not emerging as a consistent pattern in all institutions: that is not the way social change occurs. It usually comes in uneven strides. Just as an army does not move forward simultaneously on every front but must be content with a ragged battle-line whose general direction is forward, so harbingers of systems change in nursing and health care must expect uneven progress: some moving forward in leaps and bounds, others falling back into outdated policies and practices. As long as the general direction is forward, the momentum eventually will carry the laggards with the group.

Nursing's leaders need nurses who stand steady through the storm but they lose influence.

Political pragmatism

What is particularly striking about Lewis' analysis was his theory of power as applied to the historic realities now confronting the healthcare professions. Equally impressive was his perception of the role of compromise among the contending groups that a health pragmatism requires.

He begins by reciting factors that nursing leadership might well keep in mind as it prepares its strategies: "Power in decision-making is a function of knowledge, location and control of resources, as well as political skill." He describes the mechanics of power as follows: "At the turn of the century it was relatively easy to allocate decision-making power where the choices depended on special competencies which were clearly delineated by profession." Today, the boundaries blur and the competencies overlap as professionals become dependent on one another for the very knowledge critical to the decision making specific to their own domain. Moreover, the scope of problem definition today is such that choices may be seen by some that are not viewed as choices by others; thus day-to-day practice usually reconciles such differences *pragmatically.*

Someone once said that politics is the art of the possible, the two essential components of which are persuasion and negotiation. Persuasion is the art of coordinating different objectives so that people can work together to achieve a common goal.

Even when all agree on an ultimate goal, they may (make that read *almost always will*) disagree about the choice of processes and techniques to be used and the manner in which they are to be implemented. If these problems are not resolved, i.e., if all parties are unwilling to compromise, paralysis sets in. To compromise merely means "to adjust and settle by mutual agreement with concessions on both sides." Compromise is eminently possible when the conflict *means* to achieve an end rather than over the end itself. If we can agree that the goal is quality care on the continuum at the lowest cost, then the primary conflict today is over the distribution of power and the organizational techniques to be applied. If, in the struggle over the structures and the distribution of power, we lose sight of the imperatives of moral leadership—honesty, integrity, justice—ruthless men and women may prevail.

> **If we place petty concerns above the common good, we distract and disempower our leaders.**

While compromise may be eminently possible, it's likely to be extraordinarily complex and difficult. And where one or more of the parties involved is more concerned with self-advancement than accomplishment, the entire system fails.

Nurses must keep their eye on the common good but they lose perspective.

No one who calls himself or herself a leader in any profession today operates in a vacuum. Our interdependence demands cooperation, not just to survive another day, but to help make tomorrow a better day for every citizen in the U.S.A.

Nursing's leaders—in fact, all healthcare leaders—need to reach out to one another in a spirit of collegial respect, to make those compromises necessary for the development of a just and humane healthcare system.

August 1994

LEADERSHIP IN TOUGH TIMES

In every community there is work to be done. In every nation there
are wounds to heal. In every heart there is the power to do it.
Marianne Williamson
A Return to Love

In 1866, Mark Twain gave the first of what was to become a celebrated lecture series. When he came to the platform, he was so
frightened that his knees literally were knocking together. Taking a
deep breath, he said, "Julius Caesar is dead. Shakespeare is dead.
Napoleon is dead. Abraham Lincoln is dead, and I am far from
well myself." When the lecture was over, the audience had been
laughing so much they were too weak to leave their seats—and a
nation began to heal.

In 1866, Lincoln had been dead merely a year, and the nation
still mourned its lost leader. Lincoln's wit was so major a component of his leadership style that it was only fitting for humor to be
used to help heal the wounds caused by his death. In fact, Lincoln
himself once said that a good joke *gave him life*: "When I tell a
funny story," he told a friend, "...[it] puts new life into me." He
went on to say, "The fact is that I've always believed a good laugh
was good for both the mental and physical digestion."
Unfortunately, matters often were so desperate during Lincoln's
presidency that he told a staffer, "I laugh because I must not weep,
that's all, that's all."

All of this is by way of recommending to you Donald T.
Phillips' book, *Lincoln on Leadership* (Warner Books, 1993). And
this is as close to a book report as I am ever likely to write.

Few times in recent memory have been as difficult for leaders
in medicine and health care. None of us, however, have had it as
rough as Lincoln did: Seven southern states had seceded from the
union; Jefferson Davis was sworn in as President of the
Confederate States of America; and Congress refused to take any

action whatsoever to quell the rebellion—all just 10 days before Lincoln took office. By the time he was sworn in, the South had seized all federal agencies, forts, and arsenals in southern territory and controlled most of the Mississippi River, the nation's major artery for commerce. Moreover, Washington, D.C., was virtually defenseless, and the Army was in disarray as many sol-diers and officers defected to the

> **Persuade people rather than coerce them.**

cause of the South. To add to Lincoln's troubles, he was by a minority of the voters, and even his own appointees considered him incompetent. *And you think you have it bad?!*

How you treat people...

The author tackles the question: "How did this man, whose own advisors thought of him as a country bumpkin, become our most honored and revered president?" He examines Lincoln's poise and ploys and creates a very modern list of "Lincoln's Management Principles."

- *Persuade people rather than coerce them.* Lincoln believed in telling stories to persuade an audience, even if it was an audience of one. Phillips notes (p.155) that "Conversation was Lincoln's chief form of persuasion and the single most important and effec-tive aspect of his leadership style..." If the story made someone laugh, it was all the better: "Lincoln's humor [also] was a major component of his ability to persuade people...." Contemporary work in the field confirms his approach. Austin and Peters (*A Passion for Excellence*, p. 281) note: "It turns out that human beings reason largely by means of stories, not by mounds of data...." Moreover, contemporary neuroscience confirms what Lincoln instinctively knew: When you laugh, your whole attitude and per-spective change—because your brain chemistry changes.

- *Get out of the office and meet people.* Lincoln practiced MBWA (management by wandering around) long before Peters and

Waterman (*In Search of Excellence*, 1982) gave it the name. Lincoln refused to become a prisoner of his office. Nicolay and Hay, his personal secretaries, reported that he spent 75% of his time meeting with people—mostly in places other than the executive office. In 1861, the President spent more time out of the White House than in it. But meeting people isn't all there is to it: a pleasant disposition and a *positive outlook* are crucial—as is the ability to convey a sense of appreciation for what people are contributing to the endeavor.

• *Treat people with compassion.* Stories about Lincoln's compassion are legion. He was the despair of his generals for refusing to allow deserters to be shot. "If the Good Lord has given a man a cowardly pair of legs," he reasoned, "it's hard to keep them from running away with him." He was also willing to "look the other way" in order to give subordinates an opportunity to be lenient.

When General Grant asked Lincoln whether he should try to capture Jefferson Davis, Lincoln responded by telling the following story: "Out in Illinois there was an old temperance lecturer who was very strict in the doctrine and practice of total abstinence. One day, after a long ride in the hot sun, he stopped at a friend's home and asked for a glass of lemonade. When his friend asked if he wouldn't like something a bit stronger in the drink, he said, "I'm opposed to it in principle, but if a little brandy happened to slip into the lemonade all unbeknownst to me, I guess it wouldn't hurt me much." Lincoln told Grant, "Now General, I am bound to oppose the escape of Jeff Davis; but if you could let him slip out *unbeknownst-like*, I guess it wouldn't hurt me much."

Treat people with compassion.

Once a woman chided him for his leniency toward the Confederacy. "Should you not rather destroy your enemies?" she asked. "What, madam, do I not destroy them when I make them my friends?" Lincoln responded.

In *The Prince*, Machiavelli wrote, "Never make an enemy you don't have to make." Lincoln did him one better. He made his enemies his friends.

The character of the leader...

In difficult times, in rapidly changing times, in hard times, the character of the leader is more important than in other times because it can be the one source of predictability, and thus of security. One's character consists of the sum total of one's value choices.

- *Cultivate honesty and integrity.* The kids have a phrase for this today. They say, "Walk your talk." When your actions match your words, people learn to trust you even when neither of you can trust (predict) the situation. Moreover, you can believe yourself, and believing yourself is key to persuading others. Lincoln walked his talk. All his clients knew that, with Old Abe as their lawyer, they would win their case if it was fair; if not, then it was a waste of time to take it to him. One of Lincoln's secretaries reported that, after listening for some time to a would-be client's statement, Lincoln swung around in his chair and exclaimed, "Well, you have a pretty good case in technical law, but a pretty bad one in equity and justice. You'll have to get some other fellow to win this case for you. I couldn't do it. All the time while standing talking to that jury I'd be thinking, 'Lincoln, you're a liar,' and I believe I would forget myself and say it out loud."

- *Never act out of anger, fear, or vengeance.* Weak leaders make foolish and often downright cruel decisions because they act out of emotion rather than reason and compassion. Be decisive, take a strong hand, and negotiate out of strength. Pettiness and spite have no place in the successful management of any enterprise, and fear can lead you into compromises that destroy your integrity. For example, Lincoln, whose advisers often urged capitulation to the South's demands in order to avoid armed conflict, was fond of telling one of Aesop's fables:

"A lion fell in love with a woodsman's daughter, so he went to the man and asked him for her hand in marriage. Her father

replied, 'Your teeth are too long.' So, the lion had his teeth extract-
ed. When he again came back for his bride, the woodsman said,
'Your claws are too sharp.' So the lion had his claws drawn and
then he returned to claim his bride. However, the woodsman, seeing that he was defenseless, beat out his brains."

**Don't ever sell, negotiate, or compromise essentials—no
matter how badly you want something.**

Running—and changing—the enterprise

When a leader is clear and decisive, an organization is dynamic
and alive. Being decisive is not so much about giving a string of
orders as it is about setting a clear course and then putting a continuous process in place to complete the course—much like a beating heart sends blood throughout the body. To keep the process in
place:

   • *Give the greatest credit to those who do the hardest work.*
During Lincoln's last public address he said: "No part of the honor
for plan or execution is mine. To General Grant, his skillful officers
and brave men, all belongs."

When people leave your presence, have them go away thinking how great *they* are, not how great *you* are. This will inspire
them to tolerate much, and to do even more. Lincoln put it this
way, "I suppose you know that men will stand a good deal when
they are flattered."

   • *Remember that change is an emotional as well as an organizational process.* Lincoln counseled, "Understand human nature!"
People value the past if for no other reason than because it is their
history and they will mourn its loss. Kübler-Ross' stages of death
and dying apply to organizational life too. So anticipate and develop strategies to cope with denial, anger, bargaining, depression,
and exhaustion before you reach acceptance—which is the last
stage before you might actually get a buy-in. You can help mitigate
the grief response (resistance) if, when effecting change, you call
on the past, relate it to the present and use them both to link to
the future.

• *Handle unjust criticism courageously.* Anytime you make a decision, take a stand, or change anything at all, you will be criticized. Expect it, accept it, refuse to listen to those who would repeat the critical tales to you (otherwise you might be provoked to act out of anger or vengeance), but don't let it go too far. Generally, the truth is your best vindication and explanation. Tell it.

> **Any organization's most important asset is its people. Value them. Treat them well. Be honest with them. They are the ones who will bring you through the hard times.**

Provide a clear, concise statement of the direction, and justify your decision. Giving a rationale is not a sign of weakness, it is a sign of respect for the people with whom you work. Moreover, challenging a decision is not necessarily a sign of insubordination, but rather of intelligence. Don't be threatened by it; listen to what the challenger has to say; and if he's right, be flexible enough to change. If he's not, give him one of the most difficult jobs to do, but not one that will allow him to obstruct the change. Salmon P. Chase was Lincoln's Secretary of the Treasury, and one of his harshest critics. When their differences became too great, Lincoln accepted his resignation—and appointed him to the Supreme Court.

Any organization's most important asset is its people. Value them. Treat them well. Be honest with them. They are the ones who will bring you through the hard times. They are the only ones who can.

November 1994

THE GHOST OF JACOB MARLEY...

In this holiday season, when "good cheer" is a thin veneer over the ruthlessness that rules the land; when laying off competent employees of 20 and 30 years is common; when books appear proclaiming "a new era in employer-employee relationships" characterized by strict adherence to contractual obligation untainted by any sense of loyalty, one cannot help but think of Scrooge, Dickens' heartless businessman in *A Christmas Carol*. One scene in particular comes to mind: Scrooge is confronted by the ghost of Jacob Marley, his long-dead business partner. Dismayed by Marley's suffering in the afterlife, Scrooge objects "...but you were always a good man of business, Jacob." To which the ghost replies, "Business! Mankind was my business. The common welfare was my business: charity, mercy, forbearance, and benevolence were, all, my business. The dealings of my trade were but a drop of water in the comprehensive ocean of my business."

A human reflex...

Self-justification is a human reflex: everyone wants to appear to be doing the right thing, especially when such pretenses fly in the face of the obvious. Even the dishonest Innkeeper in *Les Miserables*, while in the act of robbing the bodies of the wounded revolutionaries hiding in the sewers of Paris, defended his actions: "Picking the bodies clean. Someone's got to do it. It's a public service...." A lot of people seem to be saying something pretty close to this today.

Despite the fact that in the long history of the world there has never been a generation as concerned about its emotional well-being as this one; despite the fact that whole movements are devoted to helping us face up to our deficiencies; despite all the talk about growth, very few of us are able to take an honest look at ourselves. We have thousands of ways to avoid unpalatable truths: we are callous because we have no choice; we are self-indulgent because we live only once; we are dishonest with people for "their own good." We may be impervious to, glib, or maudlin about our motives, but we are almost never utterly straight with ourselves. Most of us don't know and don't want to know.

There are, of course, good reasons for this, most of them having to do with self-defense. Rummaging about in our psyches, especially for the truth, is more than we can stand. It's our way of surviving in the world. And that being that, all our efforts to make ourselves happy invariably end up leaving us empty.

An ancient tale...

The Greek historian Herodotus told the story of Croesus (as in "rich as Croesus"). King of Lydia from 560 to 546 B.C. King Croesus had everything: power, status, money. "I am the happiest man in the world," he proclaimed.

There was at that time a great and wise lawmaker of Athens, Solon by name. So great was his fame that even centuries after his death, the highest praise that could be given to a man was to say, "He is as wise as Solon." Croesus had heard of Solon and invited him to Asia Minor as his guest. Proud as a peacock because the wisest man in the world was his guest, Croesus showed Solon all of his riches. In the evening, as the wisest of men and the richest of men were dining together, the king said to his guest, "Tell me, Solon, who do you think is the happiest man in the world?" He expected Solon to say "Croesus," but after

The messy problems of daily living often wreak havoc on our sense of adhering to the right.

thinking for a moment or two, Solon said, "I have in mind a poor man who once lived in Athens whose name was Tellus. He, I doubt not, was the happiest of all men." Intrigued, his guest asked why. Solon responded: "Because Tellus was an honest man who labored hard for many years to bring up his children and give them a good education. After they were grown and able to do for themselves, he joined the Athenian Army and gave his life bravely in defense of his country...."

Half choking on his disappointment, Croesus said, "Who ranks next to Tellus?" all the while thinking that surely Solon would say "Croesus." But Solon said. "I have in mind two young men whom I knew in Greece. Their father died when they were children and they were very poor. Their mother loved them and struggled to support them and they, in turn, worked manfully to care for her in her old age. When at last she died, they gave all their love to Athens, their native city, and served her well as long as they lived."

> **Finding moral ground in a world full of inequities, fear, and small-mindedness helps one learn to choose one's battles.**

At this Croesus became angry. "Why do you put these poor, working people above the richest and most powerful king in the world? You make me of no account, and think my wealth and power are nothing!"

Solon replied: "No one can say whether you are happy or not until you die. Neither you nor I know what misfortune may befall you, or whether your splendor will be replaced by misery."

At this, Croesus took every measure to protect what was his. Eventually, however, a powerful king, Cyrus of Babylon, attacked and destroyed Croesus' empire. As Croesus was about to be executed he thought of Solon's words and he murmured his name. Cyrus, hearing him, asked why he called out to Solon. After much persuasion, Croesus told Cyrus the tale of Solon's visit to his palace. The story so affected him that Cyrus released Croesus and treated him respectfully lest the same fate befall him. "After all," he thought, "there is no reason why we should not be merciful and kind to those who are in distress. I will do to Croesus what I would have others to do me." And that was 547 B.C.!

Of flexibility and morality...

One of the best things about such stories (historical accuracy notwithstanding) is that they condense life so that one can see the "right" answers clearly. They are not always so clear when you are living it. But we learn, we learn. The messy problems of daily living may not actually change our ideas of right and wrong, but they often wreak havoc on our sense of adhering to the right.

To thrive—even to exist—in this world (not to mention in a management or administrative post) invariably means that one learns to tolerate in oneself a certain degree of inconsistency. In a job in which *flexibility* is viewed as a cardinal virtue, one has little choice. Unbending rectitude leads to a particularly noxious form of self-righteousness that itself produces a climate inhospitable to idealism. On the other hand, *flexible* morality leads to a dangerous cynicism that accommodates almost anything in the name of self-interest. To tread the high ground between self-righteous absolutism and cynical egoism, each of us must learn to make a separate peace with reality.

This, however, is very different from "selling out." It most decidedly does not require that one desert one's sense of right and wrong; rather it requires that one *refine* it. Finding moral ground in a world full of inequities, fear, and small-mindedness, a world in which greed and unthinking cruelty frequently are encouraged—even promoted—helps one learn to choose one's battles. Each of us should know what lines she will not cross both in her personal and professional life, and those lines must remain inviolate if the human being who *is* you is to remain intact.

A few weeks ago I was talking to a nursing director whose hospital is in the midst of restructuring. A physician reported to the hospital's chief operating officer (C.O.O.) that he heard one of the head nurses complaining about the changes. The C.O.O. turned to the nursing director and said, "Fire her." The head nurse had worked in that hospital for 26 years. The nursing director sought out the head nurse and asked her for her version. After listening to her, she went back to the C.O.O. with a very different tale. The C.O.O. said, "Fire her anyway. To change the old culture we have to get rid of the old guard. She's going to be let go anyway, and this way we won't have to pay a severance."

Somehow, a trivial comment misinterpreted had become a test of her substance. She listened to the sometimes facile advice of colleagues, and she talked to herself all night about "inevitable change" and "paying the mortgage." However, in the morning she put aside self-justifications: she could not fire that head nurse unjustly. I do not have a dictionary at hand, but it doesn't matter much: one doesn't need to define the word "character" when one sees it in action.

The nursing director was discharged for insubordination, and the head nurse was laid off anyway when her job was eliminated.... *And they both have better jobs today. And they both have their self-respect.* There was no guarantee of such a happy outcome, but it's a pleasure to report that this, indeed, is what happened in this situation.

Which brings us, in a roundabout way, back to Charles Dickens and the ghost of Jacob Marley. Good business tactics, personal success, and ambition are not evil. What *is* indecent, what anyone whose values are reasonably intact *should* question, is a work situation that demands unprincipled behavior as a means to effect change or as a prerequisite for staying employed.

Many managers today are having trouble reconciling demands for making necessary changes with their ideals of common decency, loyalty, and commitment. Nurses, in particular, under intense pressure to lower costs and change delivery systems, are unprepared by experience to run roughshod over people *en route* to wherever it is administration thinks they should be going—and often find themselves in unsettling quandaries. The fastest way rarely appears to be the kindest way. Sacrificing honesty to expediency feels like betrayal of trust. Down-staffing looks a lot like reducing quality, sometimes below regulatory and even statutory minimums.

Yet, there are—and it is a measure of how cynical we have become that I need to remark on it—thousands upon thousands of people who have done very well for themselves without sacrificing one iota of integrity. Ambition and integrity are not mutually exclusive propositions. Today, more than at anytime in the last 30 years, it is essential for those in leadership positions to remind themselves that *how* one gets to the top is as important as getting there; that leaving a lousy job—no matter how fancy the title—is easier than selling bits and pieces of one's soul each day; that people are not corruptible unless they allow themselves to be corrupted.

Time-honored traditions...

I know this runs counter to accepted notions such as "Everyone can be bought." "It's a dog-eat-dog world." and "Winning isn't everything, it's the *only* thing." In fact, one of the people I asked to review this editorial said "Lousy behavior has always paid off. It's a time-honored tradition. Look at the robber barons, the privateers, sweatshop owners, absentee landlords—and a few contemporaries we can all name."

That may be so, but there are other time-honored traditions too: the traditions of Moses and Solon and Jesus Christ. The traditions chronicled by Herodotus and Dickens. The traditions celebrated at this time of the year. "God bless us every one!"

December 1994

Chapter 4

MANAGING THE NURSING ENTERPRISE

THE PERFORMANCE EDGE

Hundreds of rivets hold a 747 together. If one of those rivets fails, the airplane is in little danger of crashing. As more rivets are destroyed by metal fatigue, the chance of disaster steadily increases. Hundreds of people hold a hospital together. However, if even one of them fails, the chance of disaster is great—and steadily increases as more are destroyed by stress and fatigue.

This isn't a new phenomenon, but it is one of our growing concerns. Despite the pressure, the changes, the push to do more with less, we can't afford to fail. Nonetheless, we're coming perilously close to the performance "edge."

The Yerkes-Dodson Law

Ordinarily, the higher the goal, the stronger the drive, the greater the motivation, the more efficient the problem-solving. Indeed, this is the case, but only to a point.

A few years ago, a couple of industrial psychologists decided to test this hypothesis so they got a bunch of apes together and varied their hunger drive (motivation?) by depriving them of food for varying lengths of time. As expected, the apes' efficiency improved as they got hungrier: they even learned to work together. When pushed too far, their performance deteriorated rapidly; as their efforts repeatedly failed, they attacked one another and despaired. In either case, they got no bananas. The resulting principle, called the "Yerkes-Dodson Law" after these two researchers, is the curvilinear relationship between motivation and performance. Please note, performance improved as motivation increased until it reached a peak after which it steadily got worse. Even when encouraged, even when handed bananas, the apes could no longer cope. So, we can run along the edge of the peak, but we dare not go over that edge. The performance edge. It has two sides.

Relax, already!

Actors often comment that it's good to be a little, but not too nervous before a performance. This reflection formed the hypothesis behind yet another psychologist's research. He asked two groups of students to solve a series of problems. Members of the first group were asked for their anonymous assistance to help establish group norms for future use of the tool. Members of the second group were told that this was a test of their intelligence, morality, sense of humor and sexual potency. They were told to sign the test and, to top it all off, the researcher commented on how overcrowded the university had become as admission standards were lowered in the 60s. The results were interesting: the first group (low stress) performed significantly better on the *difficult* tasks; however, the second group (high stress) outperformed the first group on the *easy* tasks.

To explain these findings, let's go back to the apes. The apes performed poorly at both low and very high levels of stress, BUT they did worse for different reasons. When the stress level was too low, the apes just fooled around and were easily distracted. Bananas were too easy to come by to warrant close attention. When stress levels were too high, the apes persisted with an inappropriate strategy and *could not break the set* to try alternative strategies. When they met with repeated failure, they attacked one another (because they could not change the "set") and eventually despaired.

Analysis suggests that an easy task is one in which the obvious thing to do is the correct thing and a difficult task is one in which the obvious thing to do is the wrong thing. People who are driven too hard tend to persist with the obvious solution and thus do well on easy tasks and poorly on difficult tasks. Why? *Perhaps because they are too stressed to think creatively, so they just go by the rules (the mind set?).*

Creativity offers hope

Finding new solutions to difficult problems requires *creative* thinking. These are very difficult times in healthcare: to say the least, we all are stressed. In fact, highly stressed. Almost all of us have been reared and educated in the classical-rational, scientific mode of decision-making which teaches logical thinking and simply ignores creative thinking. Unfortunately, this is somewhat similar to recipes for alligator pie that begin, "First, you catch an alligator." Once you have your alligator, you can easily make your pie by following a series of clear, simple instructions. The first step of catching the alligator cannot be simply "followed": it's too complex, and too dangerous. In short, there are rules (recipes?) for logical thinking, there are no rules for creative thinking. And most of us are conditioned to follow the rules.

Preparing for serendipity

If necessity is the mother of invention, creative minds are the fathers. Although there are no clear-cut rules for creative thinking, certain factors are known to increase its probability. One we've already discussed: there must be a mutually recognized need (stress), but the environment in which the need is presented should contain as few personal risks as possible. An idea is unlikely to bud and flourish unless the environment *stimulates* (provides the need) and nourishes (reduces the risk) it.

A second, more specific, environmental factor is the chance event which offers an unexpected opportunity. Millions of people had got into bathtubs before Archimedes. Why, this particular time, did the rising of the water in Archimedes' bathtub lead to his understanding and then formulating the principle of specific gravity? He was prepared to receive it—he had pondered his problem for some time before he sat down in that tub, and he was relaxing. Serendipity strikes only the *prepared and receptive* mind. On one hand, too many people sit around in bathtubs waiting for inspiration to strike. On the other hand, too many people are so anxious-

ly diligent that they don't allow their minds to absorb the unantici-
pated. Perseverance and determination are necessary not only to
prepare the mind for a creative idea. Relaxation and personal security are necessary to open the mind to insight.

Another characteristic of creative people is *flexibility*. A familiar, if apocryphal, example is Einstein licking his finger to write on
a blackboard when he couldn't find a piece of chalk. This may be a
little thing, but it signifies a lot. To most of us, an index finger may
hold a pen or point to an example. It is difficult for us to see it as a
writing implement. Our peculiar susceptibility to mind set is the
deadly enemy of creativity.

Perseverance and flexibility—apparently incompatible characteristics—must be moderated by judgment: when do you persist
and when should you be flexible? Judgment consists of perception,
knowledge and experience conditioned by faith in oneself and others. Without judgment we persist too much as we lumber down a
dead end street—or we become too "flexible" and flit from one
street to another and get nowhere.

Beyond creativity

No one likes to be called a conformist, but few of us really relish
the notion of being a non-conformist either. Predictability is very
comforting and comfortable. In unpredictable situations, however,
it's hard to achieve. Fortunately, people are more predictable than
they are unpredictable. Therefore it really is possible to plan (predict) for the effects a creative (unpredicted) change may have on
people—and thus improve the likelihood of success.

The elements are simple: repetition, pacing, participation and
reinforcement (reward and punishment). You must display
patience and persistence as you—and *all* members of the management team—consistently present and support the change. Pace
your demands on people: don't expect them to unquestioningly
accept significant changes in the way they think or in the way they
"do" things. Start with trivial, innocuous changes and work up to
more important things. Remember that it is *never* enough to have

people merely listen and absorb; some kind of verbal or written response is essential. If someone cannot come up with an original response, give him something to copy or read or investigate and report to the group. Demand active participation at some level. Then structure the situation in such a way that responses which support the desired change are rewarded, as directly and immediately as possible.

In essence, the work experience presents a series of problems to be solved rather than a set of rote tasks to be repeated. Each employee has to solve them to remain functional and to advance. Using Maslow's hierarchy, the first (and lowest level need) is to remain employed—security is so powerful a motivator that its absence (insecurity) subsumes all other considerations. The second is to overcome fear of rejection, isolation and reprisals: to achieve acceptance and, even better, advancement. Modern management jargon refers to this as positive feedback. The third is to maintain some kind of cognitive integration—to develop a consistent outlook on life which incorporates basic values and beliefs and which supports and clarifies one's role in life. The fourth problem is to maintain a valid position before peers, to maintain friendship ties and to express concern for others. A successful organization creates a set of conditions in which collaboration with an acceptance of organizational goals leads to resolution of conflict in these areas. Progress consists of continuity and problem-solving, not conformity to routine behaviors.

You recognize, of course, the psychological principles of effect, active responding and successive approximations. The trick is to employ these while at the same time creating and nourishing an environment that welcomes serendipity. It's hard to avoid the twin horns of the conformist and the dilettante. It's even harder to know when to push and when to relax. The performance edge, for the manager, is judgment. And it's in short supply today. The rivets keep popping.

February 1989

POWER: THE TRAPS OF TRAPPINGS

George McClellan was everybody's model of what a general should be. He looked sharp and his troops looked sharp. Trouble was, they weren't doing anything but hanging around the capital. McClellan claimed that he was conducting a waiting campaign. With a superior force and ideal location, he figured that sooner or later he had to win. Meanwhile, the Confederate General Lee took every opportunity to gain ground. In total exasperation, President Lincoln sent this brief but exceedingly pertinent letter:

"My dear McClellan: If you don't want to use the army I should like to borrow it for a while.

Yours respectfully,

A. Lincoln"

Action as power

Of all the nonsense being spread around about power today (and it seems as if we're positively fixated on it—what with everything from "power breakfasts" to "power suits"), perhaps the most pernicious is the notion that power is a state of being rather than energy, status rather than dynamism, a seat rather than a vehicle.

> **If you are perceived as powerful, you are powerful.**

Knowledge as power

Take, for example, the widely accepted notion that "knowledge is power." To quote a 1930s song, "It ain't necessarily so." According to *Webster's*, *knowledge* is defined as "a clear and certain perception of something." *Thought*, on the other hand, is "the act or process of thinking" and *thinking* is "to form an idea, to conceive...; to opine; to believe; to intend..." Power isn't knowledge, it's what you *do* with knowledge. Knowledge confers potential, but that's all. Think. Have an opinion and state it. Have an idea and share it. Propose a project and do it. Use your knowledge or lose your power. Use your knowledge and increase your power. I guess that's what "use it or lose it" really means.

Position as power

When JFK was asked why he wanted to be President, he replied, "Because that's where the power is." He knew that a position of power is not a sta-

The reputation of power *is* power.

tion of arrival but rather a point of departure. Position gives opportunity. If the person who holds it doesn't capitalize on it, he soon loses both the opportunity and the position. Anyone who thinks "I've arrived" has no idea what to do with power. He (or she) won't be there long.

Power as judgment

As long as I've been telling Presidential stories, I may as well continue. Power is action, but the action must serve the mission or the results may be dire. Abraham Lincoln was criticized by his advisors for refusing to address Jefferson Davis as either "Commander" or "President" in negotiations with the U.S. government. Davis insisted, Lincoln demurred. Negotiations stalled. In a vain attempt to persuade Lincoln, his chief advisor referred to the correspondence between King Charles the First and his Parliament as a precedent for recognition of titles in a negotiation between a constitutional ruler and rebels. Mr. Lincoln's face then took on that indescribable expression which generally preceded his hardest hits, and he remarked: "Upon questions of history I do not presume to be expert. However, my distinct recollection of this matter is that Charles lost his head."

By refusing to acknowledge an assumed title, Lincoln denied the legitimacy of Davis's presidency and thus of the rebellion itself.

The union is what he sought to preserve—and *he* was its President. To yield on this point was to concede defeat. His was not the exaggerated stubbornness of the weak but rather the courage of conviction. Knowing when and what to negotiate and when and why to stand firm is power. Judgment gives direction to power which is wielded in tenacity. "Wafflers" never win.

Perception as power

According to many power brokers, if you are perceived as powerful, you are powerful. The philosopher, Thomas Hobbes, agrees. He is reported to have said "The reputation of power is power." Yes, but perception has long been recognized as an intimate interaction between the perceiver and the perceived. What and who you perceive to be powerful may say more about you (the perceiver) than them (the perceived). Psychologists have conducted experiments from the 1940s onward to explore this idea. At that time, the emphasis placed on the characteristics of the perceiver came to be called the "New Look" movement. In one such study, poor boys and rich boys were asked to adjust a circle until is was the same size as a quarter. On average, the poor boys made a circle much larger than did the rich boys, suggesting that a quarter was more important to them. Quite possibly, what you lack affects what *you* believe to be important. It can distort perceptions. It seems to me that what you think you lack could distort perception just as much. The distorted perceptions, at least insofar as "power" is concerned, could cripple you. As one famous WWII journalist, Elmer Davis, said: "The first and greatest commandment of power is, 'Don't let them scare you.'"

> Even the weak can find power in unity. Unity demands loyalty. Loyalty is one thing a leader cannot do without. And it's the one—and only—thing women lack in their struggle to gain power.

Women and power

Robert Mueller reports that he asked a Burmese man why women, after centuries of following their men, now walk ahead. He replied that there were many unexploded land mines since the war.

Today, there still are many unexploded mines in the field of leadership, but if we let them paralyze us, power—the ability to *do* something—will elude us. Leadership is action, not position. But when position and action coalesce, great changes are made. Even the weak can find power in unity. Unity, however, demands loyalty. Loyalty is one thing a leader cannot do without. And it's the one—and only—thing women (and most nurses are women) lack in their struggle to gain power. Loyalty, of course, must go two ways. If nurses want power, they need to stand behind, beside and *for* nurses. Loyalty gives power reach and durability. It magnifies its effects and gives it consistency and continuity.

No books or power lunches or power workshops or power techniques; no positions or degrees or associations; no amount of talking or contrived meetings or fancy office furniture makes one powerful. The trappings of power don't make one powerful. Knowledge and judgment and courage can and will. Action does. And loyalty makes it stick.

June 1989

Old Loyalties in the New Organization

A long time ago in *Psychiatrist's World*, Karl Menninger wrote, "Loyalty means not that I *am* you, or that I agree with everything you say, or that I believe you are always right. Loyalty means that I share a common ideal with you and that regardless of minor differences we fight for it, shoulder to shoulder, confident in one another's good faith, trust, constancy, and affection." Nurses' loyalty historically was assured principally (though not solely) through an institution's (or a physician's) demonstrated concern for patients and commitment to excellence in the delivery of their care. The places which fostered and people who gave and enabled humane and compassionate care for patients attracted nurses and won their loyalty.

Loyalty defined

Webster's New World Dictionary defines loyalty as "...faithful to those persons, ideals, etc., that one stands under an obligation to defend or support." Faithful is defined as "...true to allegiance; constant in the performance of duties or services...true, exact, in conformity to the letter and spirit."

Although in the 1770s Alexander Hamilton wrote, "The best security for the fidelity of men is to make interest coincide with duty," it wasn't until the 1970s that hospitals entered the "Age of Reason."

To this day I am shamed to recall how in 1966, I inadvertently discovered a nursing assistant eating garbage from patient trays. Tearfully, she pleaded with me not to report her for "stealing." Although an excellent worker, she earned only 35 cents an hour—

> **Do administrators or managers really believe that loyalty consists of *silent followership* and no criticism?**

less money than I made for babysitting for the neighbors 10 years earlier. The sole support of husband and child, she had no money left to pay for her own food. Who was stealing from whom?

Our founding editor, Dorothy Kelly, used to wryly observe that, in the 50s and 60s, "nurses were taught that patients were human beings, and were to be treated as human beings. Of course, they were the only people in the hospital who *were* treated as human beings..." Indeed, early attempts to organize nurses were founded as much on concern for patients and their safety as for nurses' socio-economic problems. Why? Because nurses' allegiance was still to patients and their families.

> **Those who spoke out were those who cared.**

Pushed by threats of unionization, hospital policies and structures began to change in the 1970s; rigid authoritarianism and poverty level wages had undermined employees' loyalty to the institution if not to its mission. New structures replaced the old: primary nursing, self-governing nursing staffs, participative management, self-scheduling, clinical ladders, etc., etc. And nurses once again began to associate excellence of care with specific institutions whose policies and structures melded humanitarian concern for patients with a similar concern for employees.

The more hospital administration adopted 20th century concepts, the less likely were their staffs to unionize. Indeed, few if any of the hospitals cited in the *Magnet Hospitals Study* were unionized. Nurses are seeking out hospitals with reputations for excellence, and they will be loyal to them insofar as care remains excellent and policies just. It would seem that fidelity is indeed assured when interest coincides with duty.

Has the meaning changed?

I was considerably distressed when it was brought to my notice that management researchers have been tinkering with the concept of loyalty—and *not* for the better. As far back as 1980, Kolaski and Aldrich's work refers to loyalty as "silence." Taking the hint, Rusbult et al. operationalized loyalty as a passive construct as in (ASQ34, 1989:529) "waiting patiently and hoping problems will solve themselves...saying nothing to others and assuming things will work out...quietly doing (one's) job and letting 'higher-ups' make the decisions..." According to these researchers, "...loyalty resembled entrapment in the organization more than it did supportive allegiance to the organization...the variables that predicted loyalty were, by and large, the same variables that predicted neglect...These results suggest something is seriously amiss with the concept of loyalty...Future research should operationalize loyalty as active support for the organization."

Do administrators or managers really believe that loyalty consists of *silent followership* and no criticism? If administrators and managers construe silence as loyalty and compliance as support, then they will reward the least caring, least motivated employees for neglecting their work and their organization.

Withey and Cooper, the authors of the study cited earlier, reached the conclusion that actively working to change a situation, speaking up and out about problems, is "...the only option for people who are concerned about the organization." Kay, as cited by Withey and Cooper, found in her study that those who spoke out were those who cared. Specifically, "Kay found that among the most prototypical acts of voice...were: (1) encourage discussion of issues and problems; (2) propose new ways of doing things; (3) take action on problems; and (4) make suggestions on how to improve things." This definition of "voice" is, in my opinion, the actual operationalization of loyalty, and this definition of loyalty is the only one that correlates positively with nurses' obligations to patients and to the integrity of nursing practice.

Keeping quiet, silence, in the face of problems and discontent necessarily demands disloyalty to the persons and ideals which constitute the practice and the spirit of professional nursing. To speak up, to improve, to make positive suggestions: this is loyalty.

If a healthcare organization seeks both excellent service for patients and nurses' loyalty, it must create a climate which supports both.

If the organization's commitment to excellence is genuine, speaking out is encouraged: (1) managers actually listen to employees *and* follow through, (2) therefore, employees have reason to believe that the possibility of improvement is genuine, (3) the effort required to bring about change is reasonable, (4) there is little likelihood of a punitive response, and (5) there is a possibility of personal reward. What else is required to secure nurses' loyalty? Flexible scheduling, competitive wage/benefit packages, and an atmosphere of respect. At least that's the way I read the *Magnet Hospital Study,* the report of A.H.A.'s *Commission on Nursing* and, most recently, DHHS's final report from *The Secretary's Commission on Nursing.*

> **If a healthcare organization seeks both excellent service for patients and nurses' loyalty, it must create a climate which supports both.**

The new loyalty

Are things any different as we enter the 1990s? Our institutions are undergoing wrenching changes and a whole new generation of workers are introducing an unfamiliar set of values to the workplace. For example, the desire for a good wage/benefit package and job security is counterbalanced today by a desire for more leisure time and personal advancement (mobility up and even out of the organization). Moreover, today's healthcare organizations are at once bewitched by technological advances, bothered by federal cutbacks and economic competition, and bewildered by increasing demands, especially from the uninsured. They will be hardput to keep pace with the salaries offered in business and industry in the 90s. They no longer guarantee long-term employment, and they fear that their enormous investment in continuing education and on-the-job training will only end up enriching the competition.

Where does loyalty fit in this new organization? How do today's "new" work values fit with the "old" concepts of loyalty and commitment?

Writing in the *Harvard Business Review* (November-December 1989), Elizabeth Moss-Kanter notes that "the new loyalty is not to the boss or to the company but to projects that actualize a mission and offer challenge, growth, and credit for results." The "new" motivational tools are:

1. Helping people believe in the importance of their work. "Technical professionals," Moss-Kanter holds, "are often motivated most effectively by the desire to see their work contribute to an excellent final product." Check one for nursing.

> **The new loyalty is not to the boss or to the company but to projects that actualize a mission.**

2. Agenda control—as the future of hospitals and specific services grow more uncertain, giving people more control over their professional lives becomes more important. To quote Moss-Kanter again, "more and more professionals...(seek) jobs that give them more control over their own activities and direction...Leaders give...the opportunity when they release time to work on pet projects, emphasize results instead of procedures, and when they delegate work and the decisions about how to do it." I might add that control over schedules is crucial to nurses.

3. Share of value creation incentives based on *measurable* results—like bonuses rather than raises tied to key performance targets, both for individuals and for work units. For example, a nurse may receive a healthy bonus for becoming certified or recertified in her field, and so forth. All unit personnel could receive healthy bonuses if their unit operates within its budget, quality assurance standards are maintained and patient satisfaction surveys are complimentary.

4. Learning—Moss-Kanter holds that "The chance to learn new skills or apply them in new arenas is an important motivator

in a turbulent environment because it's oriented toward securing the future...The new security is not employment security (a guaranteed job no matter what) but *employability security*—increased value in the internal and external labor markets."

5. Reputation—"The professional's reliance on reputation stands in marked contrast to the bureaucrat's anonymity." Moss-Kanter again. The old notion that the employee needs to make the boss look good must be supplemented by the boss's obligation to help his professional employees make a name for themselves. "Managers can enhance reputation—and improve motivation—by creating stars, by providing abundant public recognition and visible rewards, by crediting the authors of innovation, by publicizing people outside their own departments, and by plugging people into organizational and professional networks."

In the 1860s, Abe Lincoln's admirers loved to tell stories about him almost as much as Abe loved telling stories about them. Among the stories they told is the one about Abe's father. An old neighbor of Thomas Lincoln was passing the family farm one day when he saw Abe's father grubbing up some hazelnut bushes and said to him:

"Why, Grandpop, I thought you wanted to sell your farm?"

"And so I do," he replied, "but I ain't goin' to let my farm know it."

"Abe's just like his father," the old ones would say.

Make it work. Care about it. Make it better. That's loyalty—and the "it" can be an organization as well as a farm, and the "it" doesn't have to be forever. This concept is as applicable for the 1990s as it was for the 1860s.

March 1990

CREATING A CULTURE OF COMPETENCE

Several years ago, a *Fortune* magazine article declared, "For all the hype, Corporate Culture is real and powerful." And, for all the hype, Corporate Culture has been around for a long time. Webster's defines "culture" in various ways. "...the act of developing...the intellectual and moral faculties, especially by education; expert care and training...the total pattern of human behavior...embodied in thought, speech, action and artifacts and dependent upon man's capacity for learning and transmitting knowledge to succeeding generations..." A people, a nation, a profession, even a corporation possess cultures.

Every organization has a value system which affects decisions, styles, strategies and interpersonal relationships. What are such values, norms, and behavior patterns all about? Usually they involve:

- The basic *goals* of the organization.
- The preferred *means* by which these goals should be attained.
- The basic *responsibilities* of the member in the role which is being granted to him by the organization.
- The *behavior patterns* which are required for effective performance in the role.
- A set of rules or principles which pertain to the maintenance of the identity and integrity of the organization.

Corporate Culture is a complex concept characterized by its multi-dimensionality, i.e., it describes the implicit, invisible, intrinsic and informal consciousness of the organization which both guides and is the product of the behavior of organizational members. Moreover, the Corporate Culture of hospitals, in particular, has many layers. Each needs to be identified and evaluated in order to facilitate change. How the change is presented, what is its meaning for each subculture, what are its effects within groups and upon groups can then be evaluated and resistance as well as inter- and intra-group conflict can be mitigated or even avoided. Conflicts among subcultures can derail any plan.

In any hospital, there are at least four groups which experience the workplace very differently indeed. These groups often are so distinct that they develop unit subcultures, grouped as follows: 1) the nursing subculture; 2) the therapeutic and diagnostic subculture; 3) the support services subculture; and 4) the general and administrative subculture. In addition, the medical staff operates with the Corporate Culture but is not perhaps of the culture. The dominant Corporate Culture and these occupational subcultures meld—or collide— where strategy, vision and management style are involved. When subcultures disagree about what's important to the core business, the clash can paralyze the hospital.

Turnover studies consistently report that people who do not fit an environment tend to leave it.

By studying the degree of value consistency and value congruence as well as by dealing with specific problems on a unit or departmental basis, managers can design strategies specific to each subculture and congruent with the dominant culture. Thus, all the internal and external elements of the hospital are in line with each other and with the corporate strategy (Strategic Fit) and internal conflict and competition will be minimized.

The organizational frame of reference

The internally-induced dimensions of a Corporate Culture are translated through an organizational frame of reference (OFOR). The OFOR consists of cognitive elements, cognitive maps, reality tests, cognitive operators, codification of norms, and organizational boundaries. The *cognitive elements* consist of the basic information categories that organizational members consider valid. An organization's *cognitive maps* consist of the models by which or the standards against which organizational situations are compared and gaps or inconsistencies are labeled "problems." *Reality tests* validate information and act as "guarantors" of organizational knowledge.

Key cognitive operators order, rearrange and manage, interpret, distribute, suppress or apply information. Each element of the OFOR is affected by these key operators. *Codification* refers to the extent to which organizational expectations are written in job descriptions, policy handbooks, grievance procedures, and the like. *Organizational boundaries* refer to employees' vision of what the organization does (its role in the community, its services, etc.) and ought to do. If boundaries are too narrow, employees may resist organizational goals and/or adopt single track approaches to problems. On the other hand, if boundaries are too broad, organizational resources may be spread too thinly and strategies may become so unfocused as to lose their importance.

Leadership styles and types

The fundamental determinants of organizational behavior stem from complex interactions among and between the organization's environment, technology and structure on one hand, and the kind of people they attract, select and retain on the other hand. People who are of similar type are attracted, not only to similar jobs, but to organizations of a particular sort. Moreover, turnover studies consistently report that people who do not fit an environment tend to leave it.

Both the people and the organizations which contain them can be clustered into types based on profiles on their characteristics. As organizations evolve into maturity, the behavior of all the people in them defines the organizational culture. Initially, however, the organization's leader defines the goals to which people are attracted, selects key managers, and develops the power, performance and reward systems. In short, the leader (especially an initial leader of long tenure) designs the structure, systems, style, staff, values, skills, and strategies which collectively define the organization and determine its success or failure.

By and large, people act on the basis of the meanings things have for them, meanings that are shaped by the person's attitudes, assumptions, values and beliefs. Recent structural developmental

CREATING A CULTURE OF COMPETENCE

research suggests that most adults inhabit one of four developmental stages:

1. In the *opportunistic stage*, people tend to hold and use power unilaterally, play their cards "close to the chest," externalize blame for failure on others or situations and focus on the outside world and gaining control of it.

2. People in the *social stage* of development tend to focus on group norms and seek approval through adherence to norms.

3. *Goal-oriented* people emphasize the competent execution of rationally interrelated steps leading from strategy to implementation to extended outcome.

4. The *self-defining stage* of development is characterized by persons who are closely attuned to their inner feelings and to their outer environment.

Research indicates that most managers inhabit either the *opportunistic* or the *social* stage. By and large, self-defining leaders do not do well in organizations—unless they start them and then only during the early stages of organizational development.

"Managerial style" describes how managers manipulate power. Basically, managers choose between collecting power by joining forces and pooling resources, or competing for access to its use by pressuring or manipulating one another. "Managerial type" refers to a manager behavior profile, i.e., how he or she interacts with superiors, subordinates and with the organization.

Leader-culture fits: value-based management

The three essential components of value-based management are persuasion, negotiation and compromise. To effectively practice these arts, one must first understand that what people call "truth" is simply their interpretation of fact. People interpret facts differently because they filter them through different sets of ideals, values and experiences. Thus, they form different opinions about what the facts mean, what goals should be sought, and what decisions and actions are appropriate to reach the goals. *Persuasion* is the art of getting people to share a similar perception of the truth so that they can work together—with a minimum of time lost to frictional and transactional costs—to achieve the same goal. *Negotiation* is the art of coordinating different perceptions of the truth so that people can work together efficiently to achieve a common goal. *Compromise* is the art of identifying and trading off non-essentials so that the integrity of each party is intact as they work together to achieve mutual goals.

Even when people agree on an ultimate goal (e.g., quality care for patients at lowest possible cost), they may disagree about the choice of processes and techniques to be used and the spirit in which they are to be implemented. If these problems are not resolved, paralysis may set in. At best nothing gets done and at worst, everyone fights for his personal opinions.

Only if one can identify correctly, seek to understand the bases of differing opinions, and derive tactics which tap into commonly held values, can one begin to move the group (persons, organization, institution) off dead center. To begin, one must understand what all shades of opinion have in common. Normally, fields of opinion constitute general attitudes about the way in which power should be managed, decisions reached, goals set and met. All opinions contain intellectual and emotional elements, and all are affected by their social context: the location, time and persons (type, status and number) involved. Almost anyone can cite an "authority" to back a particular opinion and each has a personal stake not only in the expressions of his opinion, but also in its adoption by others.

> **When people agree on an ultimate goal they may disagree about the choice of processes and techniques to be used and the spirit in which they are to be implemented.**

Because most organization members agree on *overall* values and goals, the areas in which conflicts usually arise involve the techniques and processes chosen to accomplish the goals. The ability to persuade, negotiate, or compromise, as well as the ability to convey a sense of fairness and respect, depends on the managers' ability to *understand* (not just know) the bases of both employees' and the organization's values, attitudes and opinions. To the extent to which the manager can tap into—or, at least, appeal to—employees' value systems, they compliment employees' good judgment and help *vest* the employees in the organization's success.

> **Strategy is not about adaptability in behavior, but about regularity in behavior, not about discontinuity but about consistency.**

Certain leadership styles, traits, and behaviors reflect the Corporate Culture, i.e., demonstrate and model organizational values and norms and strengthen the existing culture; may be value neutral, i.e., neither strengthen nor weaken the *status quo*; or may be disparate, i.e., demonstrate values and behaviors which differ from prevailing norms or even run contrary to the norms. In either of the latter two situations, organizational conflict ensues and, depending upon how it is handled, the organization either will reject the leader or the culture will be incrementally modified. Leaders who exhibit characteristics and values which are similar to or, at least, compatible with, the dominant culture are: 1) more likely to be accepted by organizational members and 2) quite likely to strengthen the existing culture. Where a change in the culture is desired or desirable, leaders should be chosen who reflect *both* the desired culture (i.e., some of their characteristics do *not* "fit" the *existing* culture) and the existing culture, thus decreasing internal friction and increasing the likelihood of acceptance.

Strategic Fit is a situation in which all the internal and external elements relevant for an organization's success are in line with each other and with Corporate strategies. Just as some leaders "fit" better with certain cultures, so some strategies "fit" better with certain other strategies—and with the systems which are both affected by and produce these strategies. The most successful strategies for action or change capitalize on *existing* value structures. Occasionally, strategies may be adopted to *change* the *existing* value structure (culture and/or culture mores), but *to be effective* even those must have their roots in pre-existing values. Because strategies (*organizational behaviors*) demonstrate values, some strategies complement one another, some are merely compatible, and others are contradictory.

Strategy is not about adaptability in behavior, but about regularity in behavior, not about discontinuity but about consistency. Organizations adopt strategies to reduce uncertainties, to set direction, focus effort, reduce risks and define the organization. Perhaps the most significant role of strategy in organizations is to resolve the big issues so that people can get on with the details of implementation.

At rock bottom, a culture consists of a group of people who share similar values. Personal values are centrally held, enduring beliefs which guide action and judgments and provide a basic foundation for our lives. Role-related values are domain specific and consist of *both* an extension of one's personal values into the workplace *and* the shared organizational values held by the role-holders. The greater the level of shared organizational values, the greater the likelihood of "characteristic" behavior. According to Hickman and Silva in their book, *Creating Excellence*, successful corporations are characterized by: 1) employees who share an unrelenting commitment to superior customer service; 2) management which strives to hire and keep good people; and 3) employees who themselves enforce a high standard of performance. To succeed, then, the management of any hospital must share a clear strategic vision with identifiable activities, achievable time frames, and specific goals by department. Staff need to share that vision, too. When this happens, the culture supports the people who, in turn, perform with that competence upon which excellence is built.

September 1990

ATTITUDE: THE NEW POSTURE FOR THE NINETIES

"According to Richard Aldington, a famous though now deceased literary critic for the *New York Times,* his best review was never published. He explained: "In the early days of Dada (the father of surrealism), I received for review a book which contained the following poem:

A B C D E F

G H I J K L

M N O P Q R

S T U V W X

YZ

"On which I commented:

1 2 3 4 5

6 7 8 9 10

"I still think that was the most snappy review I ever wrote; but unfortunately *The Times* refused to print it."

Undoubtedly, today both author and critic would be said to have "attitude." It's considered a compliment. On an artistic/cultural level, attitude is the practice of using studied or affected techniques to dramatize one's distinctive position in one's field in an eccentric, and usually egocentric, manner. This is accepted, of course, only because this person "with attitude" has *something* (brains, talent, ability, knowledge, experience) to back it up. Elvis Presley, Mick Jagger, and Madonna all have "attitude." So do Georgia O'Keefe, Chuck Daly and Linda Ellerbee.

Politically, the roots of attitudinizing run deep, ranging from Teddy Roosevelt's "Speak softly and carry a big stick" to George Bush's "Read my lips: no new taxes." Shaped by opinion polls and TV, these kinds of sloganeering constitute the political posturings of the 90s. If they have substance, that's one thing. If they don't, perhaps ex-senator Hruska's comment during the Carswell confirmation fight does have something to be said for it. To wit: "There are a lot of mediocre judges and people and lawyers, and they are entitled to a little representation."

According to Michael Musto, who covers the night life scene for the *Village Voice*, "You go over the line when you have nothing to back it up. There are thousands of people that walk around with an attitude, but they have no creative talent. All they have is an attitude, and that's not enough to get you by."

Once the province of the artistic *avante-garde* and a few outrageous entertainers and politicians, attitude has only recently moved into the mainstream. Fueled by MTV, glitzy advertising and Bart Simpson, it has broken out of its intellectual ghetto—lots of style but little substance.

Attitude is fast becoming a buzzword for our times. One is expected to be detached, cool, even cynical. One displays the arrogance of Mick Jagger and the grungy taciturnity of Clint Eastwood all wrapped up in the sullenness of the punk movement of the 80s.

Yesterday in Wisconsin I met two nurses who were stunned because some of their newer counterparts simply would not come to work at 7:00 a.m. No call. Nothing. In New York City, several nurse managers commented that staff members called in to say "I'm not coming to work today. I'm going to the mall with some friends." Even in Minnesota, long a bastion of the work ethic, workers are refusing to do anything more when they think they've "worked hard enough for one day." These are all manifestations of attitude—as in "bad." Unfortunately, attitude has become the latest "hip" accessory of the 90s. So expect to see more of it.

> **In the male of the species [attitude] can include macho posturing; in the female, it's called bitchiness.**

Attitude can be hot or cool, natural or manufactured. Most importantly, it has its own internal consistency. According to Louis Beale of Knight News Service: "In the male of the species [attitude]

can include macho posturing; in the female, it's called bitchiness."
In the opinion of Jerry Peterson, editor of *Orbit* magazine, "An attitude is degrees of selfishness." Comments *Mother Jones's* magazine's
Ben Hampton, "It's confidence in oneself to thrust yourself upon
the world and not give a damn what people think." Whether it is
an extreme form of self-awareness or simply a theatrical guise, it's
going too far. There is a big difference between being cool and
being a jerk.

To me "attitude" sounds suspiciously like immaturity—yet
another manifestation of what sociologists are calling the Cornucopia generation. For those of you who haven't
been following the sociological literature, the Cornucopia generation consists of the Baby Boomers' children.
While there are always notable exceptions, different generations are characterized by differing values. For our
purposes, we'll confine our discussion to work values.

> **"How *could* you make out my schedule and not even consult me?"**

In the work force today we have roughly three generations:

• The children whose parents lived through the Great
Depression. We'll call them the Transition Generation (roughly
ranging from 45 to retirement age). By and large, their general attitude toward management is, "If 'they' would just get out of my way
and let me get my job done, this place would run a whole lot better." While they seek stable and equitable terms of employment,
what job satisfaction they experience comes from the intrinsic
rewards of the work itself. Management's job is to see to it that
what they need to do the job is there when they need it, and then
get out of the way. For example, Transition Generation nurses
think managers should do their own job: "When you pay me to
make out the schedule, I'll make it out. Meanwhile, it's *your job* and
good luck with it."

• The Baby Boomers, on the other hand, want to find self-fulfillment on the job—self-actualization and so forth. They range in age from about 25 to 45 years of age. They cannot imagine a world that does not want their input. Management's job is to help them grow and develop. They want to participate in decision-making and believe in decentralized structures. They want authority and accountability. They are independent and often clamor for autonomy. For example, Baby Boomer nurses want self-governing nursing staffs and self-scheduling. "How *could* you make out my schedule and not even consult me?"

• Now, we come to the Cornucopia Generation. Admittedly, they've only begun to enter the work force but already they've made their mark. It's sent McDonald's and Burger King scrambling after the "older" worker. Suddenly senior citizens find themselves in demand. Cornucopians think the workplace is there to serve their needs, and customers are there to make their lives easier. They seek dependence rather than independence: their greatest threat to their parents is "Mom and Dad, I'll never leave you!" At work, they want their managers to be understanding and accommodating, but above all, nurturing. There are now seminars for managers entitled "How to Hug Your Employee." If you hug a Baby Boomer, however, you're likely to get slapped with a suit for sexual harassment. If you don't hug a Cornucopian, he's likely to quit and go home to mommy or daddy or (if he's lucky) both of them. With the "under 25s" it's too soon to say whether they're merely kids with an attitude—i.e., whether luxury combined with prolonged education ("Mom, *everyone* takes at least five years to go through college today.") has merely extended adolescence—or whether ersatz self-confidence and selfishness will characterize a whole new generation.

Perhaps all of this is merely a fad, a kind of sociological equivalent of the hoola-hoop. Today's "style is all" mentality glorifies "marketing" over "producing" and "selling" over "servicing." If Billy Idol, Bobby Night and 2 Live Crew—today's role models?—are any indication, fasten your seat belts, ladies and gentlemen, it's going to be a rough decade.

November 1990

MANAGING IN A PRESSURE COOKER

"What does anxiety do? It does not empty tomorrow of its sorrow; rather it empties today of its strength."

Jan Maclaren
1920

Constant talk about money (or lack of it); public dissatisfaction with the healthcare system; hospital closures; disgruntled patients, physicians, administrators and personnel in general; meeting after meeting devoted to planning and/or reporting on (pick one)

- implementation of yet another change (or lack of it)
- budget (keeping within it or explaining why you can't or didn't)
- staff reductions
- reorganization (yet again)

are placing a severe strain on operations, and most especially on those managers whose job it is to assure that patients receive safe, efficient and courteous (maybe even humane?) care.

Whether you are a first-line, middle or top manager, two aspects of this situation affect you directly and very personally: you are dealing with more irritable people; and—more importantly—you must deal with your own increasing tensions.

Don't hurt yourself and don't hurt others.

Recognition

The first step is assessing your own situation realistically. Which pressures can you manage and which are beyond your authority or influence? List those over which you have control, those over which you have some control, and those over which you have no control. Put the last ones aside and do not spend energy worrying about them.

Watch your personal contacts with others—patients, peers, superiors, subordinates and so on. Make a conscious effort to identify your emotional reaction to each one. Do you emerge from the interaction feeling:
- contented?
- satisfied?
- productive?
- helpless?
- sad?
- guilty?
- hurt?
- angry?
- fearful?
- superior?
- indignant?
- let down?

In general, do you know what makes you angry? To understand your stress response, you ought to be able to describe the kinds of encounters that leave you seething. If you can recognize them, you may be able to forestall them. If not, you can certainly prepare more satisfying as well as more appropriate responses.

Prevention

Before you can lead others, you have to lead your own life. John Roger and Peter McWilliams in *Life 101* suggest the following guidelines:

• 1. Don't hurt yourself and don't hurt others.

This begins at the physical level: don't hit people, don't put things in your body that you know aren't good for you. It continues to the psychological: don't shout at others, and keep a reign on the way you talk to yourself (most peoples' self-talk is surprisingly negative, e.g., "Boy, am I stupid. How dumb can I get...etc"). And the emotional level: Don't blame others, and refuse to succumb to guilt and resentment.

- 2. Take care of yourself so you may help take care of others.

Get enough rest. Praise yourself for a job well done. Allow yourself to feel satisfaction. Consciously make an effort to enjoy the NOW of life. Treat yourself to something intellectually stimulating.

> **Take care of yourself so you may help take care of others.**

- 3. Use everything for your learning and growth.

Absolutely Everything. No matter how painful or glorious or embarrassing or funny or silly or even stupid. Easily said, but hard to do.

Cures

Psychologists Margolis and Kroes classified job-related stress into five categories: short-term subjective states (passing moods); chronic psychological responses (depression, alienation); physical health (allergies, gastrointestinal disorders, asthma, coronary heart disease); transient physiologic changes (blood pressure, PMS); work performance decrement (a simple inability to get anything done).

According to Dr. Jan Fawcett, Chairman of Psychiatry at Rush-Presbyterian-St. Luke's Medical Center in Chicago, you can cope with stress by:

- practicing relaxation and deep breathing on a regular basis
- setting time aside daily just for yourself—even if it's only a few minutes
- taking a lunch break—do not work through lunch—enjoy a relaxing meal, take a walk or exercise
- spending time with family, friends and coworkers
- being realistic about what you can and cannot do.

And maintenance

Psychologist Schacter of the University of Michigan collected reports of the experiences of prisoners in solitary confinement, of religious ascetics in retreat, of hermits and of other individuals who, by choice or circumstance, found themselves alone for long periods of time. His most consistent finding was that isolation produces anxiety. He reasoned that the need not to be alone would increase anxiety. To test his theory, he randomly divided a group of coeds in half.

> **Misery doesn't love just any old company, but only miserable company.**

The "high anxiety" group was led to believe that they would be subjected to a severe shock. The "low anxiety" group was told that they would experience a very mild shock.

As anticipated, the high anxiety group contained significantly more members who wanted to be with others. What others? Those coeds who were in a "high anxiety condition" were asked, respectively, if they wanted to be with others in the same situation or whether they would rather be with others who were waiting to see their professors. There was a marked preference to be with others in the same predicament. Misery doesn't love just any old company, but only miserable company. Moreover, only that company stewing in the same juice is truly welcome.

Conventional wisdom holds that sex is the best stress reliever. "Snuggling" ranks a close second. Laughter is the third best, and big muscle exercise ranks fourth. There may not be many studies supporting these contentions, but I surely like the approach! However, if none of these options are open to you, seek affiliation with fellow sufferers—at the very least, they'll commiserate. One way or another, we can enable ourselves to manage, and to manage well, in a pressure cooker. Who knows, a little conscious effort focused on yourself could even make it fun.

October 1991

PEOPLE MAKE THE PLACE

About 100 years ago when I was a nursing student, I lived in mortal fear that Dr. Frank Mayfield, renowned neurosurgeon and educator *par excellence*, would catch me unawares and drag me along with him on his daily rounds. For, although surrounded by an entourage of residents, Dr. Mayfield would inevitably direct his questions to whatever hapless nursing student he had caught in his clutches. Such, indeed, was my fate on bleak Monday morning.

My sufferings need not be detailed here. Suffice it to say, they were considerable. My real reason for recounting my awesome experience is to explain how I happened to hear, from the great man himself, about his encounter with a floor maid at Tewksbury Institute.

It seems that Dr. Mayfield was touring the Tewksbury Institute when, on his way out, he accidentally collided with an elderly floor maid. She was diffident and he was embarrassed. To cover the awkward moment, Dr. Mayfield started asking questions, undoubtedly in his usual purposeful and authoritative manner. "How long have you worked here?"

"Oh, doctor," the maid responded respectfully but firmly, "I've worked here almost since the place opened." "Have you, now?" he went on. "You must have seen a great many changes during that time. What can you tell me about the history of this place?"

She studied the redoubtable figure before her a moment, then slowly replied: "I don't think I can tell you anything, but I could show you something."

With that, she took his hand and led him down to the basement under the oldest section of the building. She pointed to one of what looked like small prison cells, their iron bars rusted with age, and said, "That's the cage where they used to keep Annie." By now thoroughly curious, the doctor asked, "Who's Annie?"

"Annie was a young girl who was brought in here because she was 'incorrigible'—which means nobody could do anything with her. And that girl sure was a handful! She'd bite and scream and throw her food at people. Why the doctors and nurses couldn't even examine her or anything. I used to clean up down here and I'd see them trying with her spitting and scratching at them. I was only a few years younger than her myself and I used to think 'I sure would hate to be locked up in a cage like that'. I wanted to help her, but I didn't have any idea what I could do. I mean, if the doctors and nurses couldn't help her, what could someone like me do?

> **People need their pride, and they need to know that what they did made a difference. No matter what job they hold.**

"I didn't know what else to do, so I just baked her some brownies one night after work. The next day I brought them in. I walked up real careful-like to her cage and I said, 'Annie, I baked these brownies just for you, and I want you to have them. I'll put them right here on the floor and you can come and get them if you want.' Then I got out of there just as fast as I could because I was afraid she might throw them at me. But she didn't. She actually took the brownies and ate them.

"After that, she was just a little bit nicer to me when I was around. And sometimes I'd talk to her. Once, I even got her laughing. One of the nurses noticed this and she told the doctor. They asked me if I'd help them with Annie. And I said I would if I could. So that's how it came about that every time they wanted to see Annie or examine her, I went into the cage first and explained and calmed her down and held her hand. Which is how they discovered that Annie was all but blind.

"After they'd been working with her for about a year—and it was tough sledding with Annie—the Perkins Institute for the Blind opened its doors. They must have been hurting for patients because they sent a message over here to send any of our patients who had bad eyes over to them and they'd see if they could help them. So, sure enough, they sent Annie over to the Perkins. And they were able to help her. And she went on to study and become a teacher herself...

"But that's not all. She came back to the Tewksbury to visit, and to see what she could do to help out. At first, the Director didn't say anything and then he thought about a letter he'd just received. A man had written to him about his daughter. She was absolutely unruly—almost like an animal. He'd been told she was blind and deaf as well as 'deranged'. He was at his wit's end, but he didn't want to put her in an asylum. So he wrote here to ask if we knew of anyone—any teacher—who would come to his house and work with his daughter.

"And that is how Annie Sullivan became the lifelong companion of Helen Keller.

"And when Helen Keller received the Nobel Prize, she was asked who had the greatest impact on her life and she said, 'Annie Sullivan'. But Annie said, 'No, Helen. The woman who had the greatest influence on both our lives was a floor maid at the Tewksbury Institute...' And that, Doctor, was the proudest moment of my life."

People need their pride, and they need to know that what they did made a difference. No matter what job they hold.

What an organization is...

All any organization is is a collection of people working together with certain tools to create a product or service. Sometimes they can manage even without the tools. People are your organization. Ultimately, the success of any enterprise rests on the qualities of its people. When we fail to elicit their full potential, we are impoverishing our own organizations.

> **The success of any enterprise rests on the qualities of its people. When we fail to elicit their full potential, we are impoverishing our own organizations.**

Years ago, researchers Lyon and Ivancevich reported what has become known as a landmark survey in the *Academy of Management Journal*. Using Halpin and Croft's *Organizational Climate Description Questionnaire*, they obtained data from a large Midwestern academic medical center. The questionnaire—a precursor of today's tools to measure organizational culture—was designed to elicit information on four basic measures of perceived climate:

1. Consideration—the extent to which employees are treated as individuals.

2. Rewards—both the psychological and economic compensations geared to performance.

3. Structure—the organizational relationships through which leadership operates.

4. Individual autonomy—the degree to which the climate permits people to exercise creativity, take risks, think independently and act freely.

Is what its managers do...

Translating these measures into terms to which administrators, managers and personnel could readily respond, the researchers devised key questions. The responses were then organized into eight dimensions of an organization:

1. Consideration referred to behaviors which demonstrated managers' respect for employees as human beings and their willingness to do something extra for them in human terms.

2. Trust referred to management behavior characterized by consistent demonstration of honesty in communication, follow-through on problems or concerns, and a perception of justice or fairness in recognition and reward.

3. Esprit referred to the degree to which members perceive that they achieve a significant degree of task accomplishment.

4. Intimacy referred to members' enjoyment of a congenial atmosphere: a social dimension not necessarily associated with task accomplishment.

5. Aloofness referred to formal and impersonal management behavior which demonstrates emotional distancing.

6. Production emphasis referred to highly directive management behaviors, insensitivity to communication feedback and close supervision.

7. Hindrance referred to management behaviors that did not facilitate employees' work, but rather smothered employees in petty requirements or subordinated their interests to organizational politics.

8. Disengagement referred to the behavior of organizational members who "go through the motions" to avert repercussions, do not identify with their work and lose interest in the quality of the product or service.

...which affects how people feel...

Analysis of the responses in each dimension yielded insight about what is known as "the intrinsic worth of the work itself"—cited by almost every study ever done on job satisfaction as the chief motivator, especially for professionals. How do the people, the workers, the professionals themselves experience this crucial motivator? The researchers identified four factors:

1. Belief in the importance of the work and in their ability to contribute to it.

2. Self-actualization on the job and a feeling of personal growth or progress.

3. Esteem, both self-esteem and social approval reinforced by managerial respect and recognition of their contributions. They are not just cogs in a wheel, they are not just lucky to have a job, they are special and needed and management wants them on the team.

4. Autonomy, the ability to take the initiative, and to become a participating member of the organization which, in turn, produces a sense of self-direction.

Employees are not merely acted upon. They are not denied information. They are not "protected for their own good" during hard times. They are part of the decision-making itself. Yesterday it was called participative management. Today, it's called self-governance. Whatever it's called, it adds to self-respect because it demonstrates the organization's recognition of the maturity of its employees.

...which makes all the difference

Psychologist Benjamin Schneider, writing in *Personnel Psychology* (40:3:437-451) noted that peoples' own attributes—not their external environment, technology or organizational structure—fundamentally determine how the organization behaves. Industrial and organizational psychologists have ignored this because they have been seduced into believing that the workplace determines behavior. Actually, Schneider asserts, people select themselves into and out of real organizations. Thus, the people are the setting because it is they who make the setting. This is true of all personnel, but it is particularly true of leaders and professionals. Just as form follows function, so people make the place.

...And all the difference in the world between success and failure.

In our business, that means living or dying or finding something to live for. Nurse initiative, ingenuity, knowledge and skill can make an enormous difference in the lives of real people who live in the real world. That's what the floor maid at the Tewksbury Institute was proud of. That is what nurses—usually in far more sophisticated ways—do every day.

In fact, everything nurses learn, all the skills they develop, are meant to make a difference. And they do. Nurses are people who make a difference. I am so grateful to be one of you.

May 1993

EMPOWERMENT: ON EAGLE'S WINGS

A baby eagle fell from his nest high up in the craggy mountains. He broke his wing in the fall and it was very cold—and dangerous: predators lurked all around. Luckily for the eagle, a man named Lyndon was mountain climbing that day. He found the injured eaglet and had pity on him. He scooped the eagle up, took it home, set its broken wing and put it outside in the chicken yard, for Lyndon owned a large farm with many chickens and chicken coops.

By this time, the little eagle was very hungry but he did not know what, no less how, to eat with this strange tribe of birds. But he was pretty smart, so when he saw Lyndon throwing chicken feed, and the chickens pecking away at it, he started pecking, too. And so it came to pass that the young eagle ate the grain and his wing healed and he grew larger and stronger. Yet still, he pecked away at the grain in the chicken yard. He seemed to have forgotten that he is an *eagle*.

One day Lyndon's friend, Hillary, came to visit and she saw the eagle pecking away at the grain in Lyndon's chicken yard. And she said to Lyndon, "What's that eagle doing in your chicken yard? He belongs out in the wild, soaring through the mountains, consorting with other eagles—not pecking away at grain in a chicken yard!"

"Look," Lyndon said, "that eagle knows a good thing when he sees one. He was cold and dying in the mountains when I took him down to my farm, healed his wing, and gave him food." Hillary was troubled, and she asked, "Lyndon, did you ever even try to teach your eagle to fly?" Lyndon responded, "He stays here because I gave him what he wants: free grain and a warm coop. He wouldn't fly away from here if he could!"

"Oh yeah," Hillary said, "I bet you ten bucks I could teach your eagle to fly away and be free."

"You're on," said Lyndon.

So, Hillary went out into the chicken yard and picked up the young eagle and carried it to the top of the barn. She told him,

"You are an *eagle*, not a chicken. You can fly into the air, over the farms into the mountains. You can be *free*."

The young eagle heard what Hillary said and he was excited. But then he looked down into the chicken yard and saw the chicken feed and the warm coops, and he heard the hens clucking. Then he remembered what had happened to him the last time he had been up so high—and his wing hurt just thinking about it. No matter how much Hillary encouraged, persuaded, and begged, the eagle would not fly. And, besides, he didn't know how, anyway.

Finally, Hillary had to carry the eagle back down to the chicken yard. Lyndon pocketed his $10 and Hillary's last sight was of the eagle pecking grain amidst the hens.

But Hillary did not give up. The next day she was back again with another plan, and this time she bet Lyndon $50 she could get the eagle to fly away. Lyndon said, "Sure, Hillary, I *like* making money."

At that Hillary strode into the chicken yard, picked up the eagle and took him to her car. Then Hillary drove the eagle up into the mountains and spent the whole day teaching that eagle how to spread his wings and flap them. She encouraged the eagle and complimented it. Near sunset, she took the eagle to the top of a mountain and she said, "You *are* an *eagle*. And now you *can fly* and be *free*." And she let the eagle loose, and the eagle stretched its wings and flew into the air and it soared and swooped. It felt the rush of wind through its feathers and it knew joy for the first time in its life.

As the eagle swooped down the side of the mountain and over the plains, it saw the familiar outline of Lyndon's farm. It saw the chicken coops, and remembered the grain. And the eagle was hungry after all this work...

By the time Hillary drove back down the mountain and pulled up to Lyndon's farm, the eagle was in the chicken yard, pecking away at the chicken feed.

Lyndon grinned from ear to ear as he pocketed Hillary's $50, but he was too much of a gentleman to say, "I told you so."

Hillary felt pretty sorry for herself, and she started blaming the eagle for acting like a chicken, refusing freedom when it was offered, and costing her so much time and money. She brooded and whined for several days, but then her brain kicked into gear. It took her a whole week to devise and test her new plan. However, by Saturday morning, she was ready. She hopped into her car and drove back to Lyndon's farm. She bet Lyndon $100 that she could teach the eagle to fly and be free. All Lyndon said was, "There's one born every minute," and started figuring out how he'd spend his winnings.

Hillary stealthily entered the chicken yard, put a hood over the eagle's head and spirited him out of the coop and up into the mountains. As the sun rose, she showed the eagle other nests, and they watched adult eagles hunt and dine and feed their young. As the sun reached high noon, Hillary and eagle watched his peers fly and sun themselves. In the afternoon she showed the eagle the beauty of his life and homeland, and she taught him again how to fly. She encouraged the eagle to hunt, and most of all, she kept reminding him, "You are an eagle. You are an EAGLE!"

On the second day in the mountains, she told the eagle the story of the chickens. "Chickens," Hillary said, "are only good for three things: laying eggs, hatching chicklings, or selling to the slaughter house. You can't lay eggs, and you'll never hatch a chickling." The eagle got the idea. As I said, he is a pretty bright bird. At any rate, by that evening, the eagle and Hillary traveled together to the top of the highest mountain where she bade the eagle goodbye. And, with barely a flip of his tail feathers, the eagle took off and soared into the night. And he never looked back—and he *never* ate chicken feed again. For he was an EAGLE and he knew it!

The parable of the eagle...

Anecdotes are stories with points. They are tools—nail sinkers—to drive home arguments fully. In their oldest form, they were known as parables. By means of them, the Greek slave Aesop told stories that embodied profound teachings. The prophets and sages of all ancient religion and wisdom employed the simple, effective parable. "I will liken him unto a wise man who built his house on a rock..." "There went out a sower to sow..." "A certain man had two sons..."

A good story has many layers of meaning, and many interpretations. The parable of the eagle is no exception. To my mind it represents what *empowerment* is all about; whether it is the empowerment of the disenfranchised, the poor and the wounded. Or whether it is about the empowerment of a nursing staff, the health-care system or a whole nation.

It (empowerment) isn't easy. Telling the eagle to fly wasn't enough.

It isn't easy. Changing the eagle's environment and even teaching him how to fly wasn't enough.

It isn't easy. You have to start at the beginning and recreate an attitude in a new environment.

It's tough on the eagle, too. The eagle was frightened: he had been hurt. The eagle knew the old, safe ways of pecking and free grain and a warm nest. And he could have that with no effort! It was hard for the eagle to believe that the easy way sooner or later would destroy him. And it was really tough on the eagle when Hillary blamed him for being what he'd been taught to be all his life.

No. It isn't easy to empower others—or, for that matter, to be the ones *being empowered* either. Don't give up. Don't whine too much when things go wrong. Keep dragging the eagles out of the chicken coop. And know that empowerment is going to cost money, time and effort.

Freedom isn't easy, and it isn't for everyone.

Risk isn't easy, and it isn't for everyone.

Abraham Lincoln was often the despair of his generals because of his lenient treatment of cases where soldiers were absent without leave. "If the good Lord has given a man a cowardly pair of legs," Lincoln reasoned, "it is hard to keep them from running away with him."

Don't blame the chickens for being what they are. It's unfair—and it's a waste of time. But never give up on the eagles. They *can* fly—and they *will*. Heal them. Give them a reason. Teach them *who* they are. Change their environment. Show them how. Again. And again. *Then*, throw them off the mountain.

June 1993

BLESSED ARE THE FLEXIBLE...

Earlier in this century, when the architect Frank Lloyd Wright was
at the peak of his profession, he designed and built a cluster of
office buildings around a central green. When the construction was
complete, the landscape crew asked him where he wanted to place
the sidewalks. He responded, "Don't put in any sidewalks just yet.
Plant grass solidly between the buildings, and we'll know where to
put them soon enough." The buildings were rented and as people
moved in and out and all about, paths of trodden grass laced the
lawns between the buildings. These paths turned into gentle curves
and were sized according to traffic flow. When Mr. Wright saw
them, he said, "Pave the paths." Not only were the paths graceful,
but they also responded directly to users' needs. *He adapted changes
to the natural patterns of the people affected by them.*

Perhaps the greatest problem in the days ahead will not be
AIDS or aging or healthcare reform. It probably will be the acceptance of change *as a way of life.* And the key to successfully managing change just might lie in Frank Lloyd Wright's approach to it:
accommodate the natural pattern of those affected by it.

Change as torture?

In 1532, Machiavelli wrote, "There is nothing more difficult to take
in hand, more perilous to conduct, or more uncertain in its success, than to take the lead in the introduction of a new order of
things...The innovator makes enemies of all those who prospered
under the old order, and only lukewarm support is forthcoming
from those who would prosper under the new...because men are
generally incredulous, never really trusting new things unless they
have tested them in experience."

Actually, Machiavelli *understates* the difficulties you face in
introducing change. Even those who have not prospered under the
old ways of doing things want to cling to the familiar! Almost 30
years ago a Canadian neurosurgeon conducted some experiments

that revealed the intensity of this problem: when people are forced to change viewpoints, the brain undergoes a series of changes that are biochemically similar to those experienced by individuals who are being tortured. Is it any wonder that people resist change, *particularly when it is forced?*

Even Winston Churchill, one of the most daring men in the 20th century, said, "When it is not necessary to change, it is necessary not to change." He wanted to conserve what had proved effective in the past; he was prepared to strike out in new directions only if the old ways had to be abandoned.

The manager's role...

And what is a problem for the individual becomes a problem for the organization. We recently polled a sampling of *Nursing Management's* readership and every response had to do with effecting change, managing change, overcoming resistance to change and surviving change. As one nurse manager put it, "When I go to bed at night, I don't know whether or not my job will have become obsolete by morning. Change is a daily thing with us."

Between our reluctant departure from the womb (resisting change from the start!) to our equally reluctant departure for the tomb, we live under a pro tem set up that is constantly shifting— like a ship at sea. And, like an ocean liner, we need a gyroscope— an instrument *that adjusts the ship to the natural rhythm of the sea and the rise and fall of the winds*—to keep us on an even keel. The manager's role; *i.e.* to be a gyroscope, maintaining balance and perspective, adapting changes to suit the pace and personalities of staff whenever possible. That is, like a ship, the organization has a goal, but it will not reach its goal unless *it adjusts to the natural patterns of* the personnel who are the organization. Just as the organization expects employees to be flexible, so it also must be flexible.

The good old days...?

Years ago, as a student of philosophy, I was "led down the garden

path" by an ancient Greek by the name of Heraclitus who said:
"What is, is. And what is not, is not." That seemed an eminently
reasonable dictum to me, until Heraclitus' inexorable logic continued: "Therefore, what is always was and always will be, and what
is not never was and never will be." Slowly, step by step, he led me
to what was to become his most famous and most often quoted
"law", i.e., "The only constant is change." Your institution is going
to change. Your job is going to change. The people around you are
going to change; your environment, your tools of living, your community is going to change. Society, culture and technology are
going to change. (And I might add, while thumbing my nose at
Heraclitus, *not* always for the better.)

Not, let me hasten to add, that I am against change. When I
find myself longing for the "good old days," I read over a list of
"Rules for Nurses" posted in 1905 by a hospital in the northeast:

1. Nurses will fill lamps, clean chimneys and trim wicks.

2. Each nurse will fetch a bucket of water for scrubbing and a
scuttle of coal to stoke the fire before beginning her rounds.

3. Each nurse is to record her observations carefully and legi-
bly. She must make her pens carefully, and she may whittle nibs to
her individual taste.

4. The nurses will be given one evening off each week for
courting purposes, or two evenings if they go to church regularly
and the superintendent of nurses gives her approval.

5. After 13 hours of work, the nurses should spend their
remaining time reading the Bible and other good books.

6. Every nurse should lay aside from her pay each week a
goodly sum of her earnings for her declining years so that she will
not become a burden on society.

7. The nurse who has performed her duties faithfully and
without fault for five years will be given an increase of $.05 per
day in her pay, providing the hospital's situation permits.

I do not know about you, but reading that list makes the
thought of change warm the cockles of my heart.

The nurse as change agent

Regardless of how individual nurses may react to change, by the very definition of their role, nurses are change agents. That is, a nurse is brought into a situation precisely because the patient's *status quo* is not acceptable. As perceived by the patient, the role of the nurse is to bring about a desired change. Moreover, it is through observation and analysis that the nurse is expected to bring about that change.

Ultimately, what really counts is your ability to understand how you relate to the change process—be you staff nurse or manager. Over 100 years ago, Florence Nightingale said: "What the nurse has to do is to put the patient in the best frame possible for nature to act upon him." To determine what needs to be done, how quickly it can be done, what constitutes "the best frame possible," and who (patient or nurse) ought to do what are matters for critical analysis. Over 30 years ago, Hildegard E. Peplau (who was proclaimed a *living legend* by the American Academy of Nursing last fall) suggested just how/when this analysis is done: "The nurse is a participant observer in most relationships in nursing. This requires that she use herself as an instrument and as an object of observation at the same time that she is participating in the interaction between herself and a patient or a group. The more precise the nurse can become in the use of herself as an instrument for observation, the more she will be able to observe in relation to performances in the nursing process."

Only on the basis of such critical self-examination can clinical nurses be effective "gyroscopes" for patients, matching interventions with the patients' natural patterns. And only on such a basis can nurse managers be effective "gyroscopes" for the organization, matching change with the natural pattern of patient, staff and institution.

Blessed are the *flexible*, for they shall *change* the earth!

March 1995

Chapter 5

HEALTH CARE REFORM: POWER AND POLITICS IN HEALTHCARE

ECONOMIC COMPETITION: HAS THE "SOLUTION" BECOME THE PROBLEM?

According to Webster's, competition is "the act of seeking to gain what another is seeking to gain at the same time and usually under (or as if under) fair or equitable rules and circumstances." Webster's goes on to note that competition also may be defined as "a market condition in which a large number of independent buyers and sellers compete for identical commodities, deal freely with each other and retain right of entry and exit from the market."

In the past, what competition there was among hospitals usually was confined to medical technology, quality care and reputation. Economic competition was discouraged by regulatory and tax measures that encouraged employers to provide comprehensive health insurance, that increased access to the disadvantaged and that discouraged price-competitive behaviors among providers.

Faced with an aging population, rising social expectations and technological possibilities, and sky-rocketing costs, business and government alike pushed for economic competition among hospitals by fixing prices through contract, capitation and/or medical diagnosis.

• Herzlinger, writing in the *Harvard Business Review*, notes that "entrepreneurialism ran rampant and forgot sound management principles.... The usual reason for failure: the entrepreneur's obsession with financing and fixation on marketing... [In doing so, they neglected] four key areas: administration of operations, management of human resources, management control systems, and the formation of a management philosophy." Among the results: a G.A.O. study indicates that marketing and reorganization accounted for one-third of the increase in hospital costs from 1982 to 1987. Moreover, quality of care is "notoriously erratic" and inflation rates are considerably above those found in the general economy.

• Robinson, a health economist writing in the *Milbank Quarterly*, warns policymakers against "...rushing headlong down a deregulatory path guided by an analytic model increasingly abandoned by its original components." A proliferating number of economists argue that "intelligently designed regulations can improve market performance and increase social welfare." In short, a price-competitive market does not seem to have produced cost-effective organization or efficient delivery. That's putting it mildly: while one in eight American dollars goes for healthcare, as many as one in five Americans is medically indigent.

• Dougherty, writing in the *Hasting's Center Report*, notes that "the lack of a severity of illness index, combined with an inequitable distribution of the most ill patients, creates an incentive to avoid the very patients who need hospital care." He could have added that pressure on hospital margins makes it difficult for even the most charitably inclined to open their doors to the indigent. Some hospitals don't even want to take too many Medicare and Medicaid patients. Everyone competes for the "healthy," insured patient who needs an over-reimbursed procedure.

> **Professionals and corporate executives lost sight of the common good.**

What went wrong? With 90 percent of the nation's HMOs in financial straits, and a shocking number of U.S. hospitals in deep waters financially, government and business alike are looking at control of physician practices (admitting patterns, treatment regimens, etc.). So deep is the concern about physician conduct that Congress is actually considering "ethics legislation" that attacks physician ownership or investments in home health agencies, long term care facilities, pharmacies, and durable medical equipment companies to which they send or refer patients. It should come as no surprise to anyone that studies prove that physicians inevitably refer more patients to their own companies.

What went wrong? Administrators relied on financing "fixes" rather than strong cost accounting measures. Paper gains rather than operating revenues made bottom lines look good—temporarily. Marketing "experts" held out unrealistic promises of profitability and market share which financially strapped or organizationally emasculated operations people could not deliver.

What went wrong? Healthcare *consumers* (and this includes both the "buyers" and the "recipients" of care) 1. do *not* enter the acute care market at will; 2. do not leave this "market" at will; 3. are constrained by the depth and breadth of information provided to/for them, by the lack of outcome measures, by often critical time factors, and by the services available to them locally.

Healthcare *providers* 1. do *not* provide identical services; 2. are burdened by oppressive state and federal regulations/constraints; 3. are constrained by heavy capital and labor costs; and 4. have little control over medical staff decisions regarding the allocation and use of their human and material resources.

Such constraints on *both* providers and consumers make it difficult indeed to imagine a competitive "free market economy" in healthcare. In fact, it's a rather sick joke.

Why did things go wrong? According to Duke University President Brodie, in driving for their own personal success, professionals and corporate executives lost sight of the common good. He castigates those who believe that profit-oriented models *alone* can fill social needs. Social cooperation is a *sine qua non* for success in human services.

It seems to me that efforts to reform the healthcare system did not fail of their own accord. Regulatory systems did not fail of their own accord. Regulatory initiatives were *not* intelligently designed. Moreover, many people sabotaged the system—even more simply weren't equal to the radical changes in *perspective* and *behavior* required. *For too many key actors had too much vested in the "old" system in which they had achieved both wealth and power to help change it.* Nonetheless, the healthcare system *did* change—and growing numbers of reports indicate that the change was *not* for the better.

If we are going to create a better system, we—all of us in health services—had better start becoming part of the SOLUTION rather than part of the problem.

May 1989

Rube Goldberg and The Great American Healthcare System

An old man in a wheelchair robbed a bank. It was near the end of the month and he'd run out of money...and he'd run out of his medications, too. So he went to the bank to withdraw his savings—he'd thought he'd saved enough to cover the costs. But what with service charges and the like, he was $17 short. So...he threatened to blow up the bank unless they gave him $17. The alarm was sent out and police were everywhere. I ought to know: I was stuck in the traffic jam.

Only that morning, while reading the editorial pages in our local newspaper, I'd come across a report on a court case. A man, irreversibly comatose, had been removed from all means of life support at his family's request. A public interest group, outraged by this alleged violation of his rights, sought a court order to resume life support. It was granted. The daily cost of his care is about $1,000. No one had to rob a bank: the public pays the bill.

Just two weeks ago, I talked to a friend who mentioned that she was collecting money for a neighbor. He has cancer—and his insurance ran out and he needed $2,000 to pay for his last two chemotherapy sessions.

Another friend's son is uninsured because his employer's health insurance won't cover him because he was born with hemophilia.

What kind of healthcare system have we got? We throw millions (for all I know, billions) into the "treatment" of the irreversibly dying and abandon those who could actually live with just a little help. Something is very wrong here.

In March, when Senator Ted Kennedy keynoted the 38th National Health Forum, he noted:

- 33 million Americans are medically indigent—more or less permanently.

- another 36 million people will have no insurance coverage for significant periods of time this year

EXHIBIT I

COMPARISON OF SYSTEMIC REFORM PROPOSALS

Coverage	Benefits	Administration	Quality
Kennedy/Waxman			
Requires employers to cover all full-time workers; expanded Medicaid program covers low-income and other uninsured persons.	Provides hospital, physician, prenatal and well-baby, and some mental health benefits; maximum out-of-pocket costs are $3,000 per family.	Maintains administration by employers, private insurance, Medicare, and Medicaid.	Recommends development of clinical practice guidelines and use of peer review organizations.
Enthoven/Kronick			
Employers cover full-time workers; employers pay tax on behalf of uncovered workers who would receive coverage through public sponsor; Medicare and Medicaid remain intact; uninsured obtain coverage through public sponsor.	Includes benefits offered under HMO Act, possibly with some restrictions; out-of-pocket costs cannot exceed 100% of insurance premium.	Maintains administration by employers, Medicaid, and Medicare; encourages states to develop public sponsor to ensure coverage for all those not covered by above groups.	Recommends risk-adjusted monitoring of outcomes based on uniform database.
Health Security Partnership			
All non-Medicare beneficiaries covered by a single program, administered by state agencies that serve as intermediaries with qualified plans; Medicare integrated with the Health Security Partnership.	Provides hospital and physician, prenatal and well-baby, inpatient prescription, diagnostic test, mental health, substance abuse, rehabilitation, and phase-in of long-term care benefits; maximum out-of-pocket costs are $2,500.	Eliminates employer health benefit and Medicaid administration; sets up state insuring agencies to serve as intermediary between all state beneficiaries and health plans.	Establishes National Advisory Commission on Technology Assessment to assess appropriateness of care, state standards for length of stay, etc.
Heritage Foundation			
All individuals required by law to obtain basic catastrophic health insurance coverage.	Does not specify benefits that must be included in a catastrophic package; long-term care covered for low-income persons; cost sharing varies by income.	Eliminates employer health benefit administration; benefits administered through private insurance companies; restructures Medicaid and Medicare.	Does not discuss specific quality initiatives.
National Leadership Commission			
Employers cover employees or pay tax for employee coverage by state UNAC programs; uninsured and all low-income persons, including non-long-term care Medicaid beneficiaries, covered by UNAC; Medicare remains as is.	Does not stipulate benefit package; suggests that benefits be decided in public forum; recommends inclusion of mental health, preventive, and prenatal care; maximum out-of-pocket costs are $3,000 per family.	Maintains employer health benefit and Medicare administration; sets up state UNAC programs to ensure coverage for all uninsured and current Medicaid eligibles receiving acute care.	Establishes National Quality Improvement Initiative to develop and disseminate information about quality of care.

Financing	Cost	Cost Containment
Employers pay 80% and employees 20%; employers pay less for those working 17.5 to 25 hours per week; those with sufficient income buy into Medicaid; low-income persons are covered by Medicaid.	Estimates range from $18 billion to $100 billion per year for employer costs; public program estimates being prepared	Managed care
Employers pay 80% of average cost of health plan; employees pay 20%; employers pay tax of 8% on first $22,500 in wages for uncovered employees; self-employed, retirees, and uninsured with sufficient income pay 8% tax on adjusted gross income (AGI); low-income persons up to 150% of poverty line are subsidized.	Net additional cost estimated at $15 billion, a one-time cost increase	Managed competition; partial elimination of employee tax exclusion for employer's health insurance contribution
Combination of employer and employee payroll taxes, general revenues, "sin" taxes, and other taxes that states may designate; all revenues paid into state Health Security Partnership funds.	$31 billion per year	Federal expenditure growth limited by economy's growth; state and territorial budgets; use of physician relative value scale, prospective payments for hospitals
Individuals pay the cost of health insurance; tax credits available; low-income persons receive subsidies.	Cost not estimated	Consumer-driven cost containment with use of extensive cost sharing
Employers pay 75% and employees 25%; employers not providing coverage pay 9.68% on first $45,000 in wages; employees pay 2.04%; for low-income uninsured, employers pay 0.68% and employees 0.66% of AGI up to $45,000.	$15 billion to $20 billion per year	Utilization control mechanisms; provider information on efficacy of procedures; preferred provider organization and HMO contracting; malpractice reforms; provider reimbursement negotiations

EXHIBIT I

COMPARISON OF SYSTEMIC REFORM PROPOSALS

Coverage	Benefits	Administration	Quality
Physicians' Proposal			
Includes all Americans in a single national plan administered by states; eliminates Medicare, Medicaid, and private insurance.	Includes all medically necessary care, including acute, long-term, rehabilitation, dental, occupational health, and prescriptions; no cost sharing.	Eliminates Medicare, Medicaid, and all private insurance; establishes state-administered programs in accord with national guidelines.	Does not discuss specific quality initiatives.
Stark MediPlan			
Requires employers to provide comprehensive benefits through private health insurance or HMOs; requires nonworking individuals not covered by employer plans to purchase these same benefits; public program similar to Medicare covers all low-income and other uninsured persons.	Provides all current Medicare benefits and adds first-dollar coverage of prenatal and labor and delivery services, well baby and well child care, nursing home care, full home and community-based benefits; restores 180-day Medicare skilled nursing facility benefit; maximum out-of-pocket costs are $2,000 per individual and $3,000 per family.	Maintains administration by employers, private insurance, and Medicare.	Does not discuss specific quality initiatives beyond quality assurance mechanisms currently in Medicare.
Pepper Commission			
Phases in health insurance coverage through a combination of employment-based coverage and a public plan; also phases in coverage for home and community-based care and protection against impoverishment for those in nursing homes.	Includes basic hospital and physician services, limited mental health benefits, and preventive services; maximum out-of-pocket expenses are $3,000 per person or family.	Federal government would administer public plan, but states can choose to do so; long-term care portion administered by states, subject to federal guidelines	Calls for a national system of quality assurance that includes national practice guidelines and standards; suggests development of a uniform data system to serve as the basis for quality assessment.
AMA Health Access America Proposal			
Extends access to affordable health insurance coverage to all the uninsured.	Does not define specific benefits package but suggests that individuals be able to choose coverage beyond a basic benefit and additional coverage should not be mandated by law.	Maintains administration through existing mechanisms of private insurance, Medicare, and Medicaid.	Calls for expanded federal support for medical education, research, and the National Institutes of Health; also suggests development of professional practice guidelines.

Financing	Cost	Cost Containment
Financing through progressive taxes.	No additional expenditures if cost-containment measures adopted	Global budgets and expenditure caps set at percentage of GNP
Employers pay 80% and employees 20% of premium through payroll tax of 50 cents per hour; self-insured pay entire premium; sliding-scale subsidy for working Americans and full subsidy for nonworking Americans with incomes up to 200% of the poverty level; public program financed through progressive 4% health tax on personal (and corporate) gross income over $16,000 per year.	Net federal costs of $120 billion annually on full implementation in seven years	Uses current Medicare policies; prospective payment for hospitals and nursing homes, RBRVS and volume performance standards for physicians
Does not address financing specifically, but suggests progressive financing.	Estimated at $66.2 billion per year on full implementation	Suggests consumer cost sharing, medical malpractice reform, managed care, and the extension of Medicare payment rules to the public program
Suggests individual and employer tax contributions to strengthen Medicare's financial base; does not mention additional specific measures.	Does not provide cost estimate	Suggests encouraging patients to make cost-conscious decisions; also suggests that RBRVS for physician payment under Medicare be used to rationalize physician payment

- 60 percent of insured Americans are underinsured.

We, the people of the United States, spent 660 billion dollars on healthcare in 1990 (that is about $2,640 for every man, woman and child) and yet one million of us were turned away from needed (not necessarily life-saving) healthcare...and four out of every 10 children got no immunizations. Something is very wrong here.

A culture of character...

Mr. Louis Sullivan, Secretary of the Department of Health and Human Services, during his luncheon address, called on all Americans to develop a "Culture of Character" to solve the healthcare crisis in this country. If Americans would stop drinking (alcohol) and smoking (anything) and practice safe sex and lose excess weight and exercise regularly ("Americans know they only have to exercise 20 minutes, three times a week to improve their health, and they don't do it!")—none of which *costs any money*—they would be healthier. If women would spend more time at home with their children, our drug problem would be significantly reduced. What this country needs is a good old-fashioned dose of character...which sounds suspiciously like "blaming the victim." Maybe the man who needed $17 wouldn't have gotten sick when he got old and the other man wouldn't have gotten cancer and the boy would not have been born with hemophilia if they had "character"...but I doubt it.

Meanwhile, tobacco subsidies are unlikely to be cut, clean air legislation faces an uphill battle, and the incidence and prevalence of infectious disease (tuberculosis, pneumonia, etc.) are increasing rapidly as homelessness and malnutrition attack the very foundations of health. Something is very wrong here.

Prevention *is* preferable to and cheaper than treatment. But prevention is not possible nor will treatment be financially feasible until we have some sort of universal access to at least basic care for all Americans. And I must add that *even* then, to quote New York City's health commissioner Woodrow A. Myers (and New York has a universal access system!): "We can't expect to get results from

21st century, high-tech medicine when people live in 19th century conditions."

Congressional proposals

With at least half of all Americans uninsured or underinsured, the political pressure is building. From out of the mouths of insurers, employers, labor and industry, clergy and politicians, comes a call—nay, a demand—for radical reform of the healthcare system. Eleven proposals (nine of which are outlined in Exhibit I) developed within the past three years have the same goal—to provide all Americans with health insurance coverage—but suggest very different means to achieve that end. One thing seems sure—we will have some kind of universal coverage. And reimbursement will be tied to both volume and outcomes. And lower tech, less invasive diagnostics and therapeutics will proliferate...but not yet. Upon America's entry into World War II Winston Churchill remarked: "You can always count on Americans to do the right thing—after they've tried everything else." I guess that's still the case.

Rube Goldberg is a cartoonist so famous for his complicated "inventions" that he actually made the dictionary. "Rube Goldberg, 1) having a fantastically complicated, improvised appearance, 2) deviously complex and impractical." I can think of no better phrase to describe today's healthcare system. To paraphrase Rube himself (from the foreword of his book, *How to Remove the Cotton from a Bottle of Aspirin*): As we move forward along the regulation-strewn path to universal coverage we become more and more aware of its general theme. DO IT THE HARD WAY. Do *not* look for the final resolution until you have followed each stage in its tortuous advance toward completion.

Within three to eight years we will have a universal access system, and we'd better start looking and following—and *influencing*—its tortuous advance. The future of our profession, our practice, and our patients depends on it.

May 1991

THE REVOLUTION BEGINS ANEW...

Once Congress passed the DRG legislation in 1982, it looked as if the revolution had come. Hospitals downsized and diversified their operations, stratified "products," and "marketed" new ones. The 80s saw the growth of hospital chains, outpatient surgeries—and medical indigency. Nevertheless, despite everyone's good intentions, we paved the road to hell. Costs skyrocketed and access plummeted. The revolution fizzled.

So, what now? Congress—unwillingly and unhappily—is contemplating no fewer than eleven proposals for radical change in the U.S. healthcare system. Not one will be adopted this year as drafted—and I don't think any one of them will be adopted even if amended. Moreover, the U.S. will not adopt either the English or the Canadian system. Certainly, we will not nationalize the healthcare industry. I think we will adopt our own peculiar brand of quasi-socialized system that will parallel our quasi-entrepreneurial system as closely as possible.

For a number of years, the Federal government has been backing out of directly delivering service itself and, at the same time, pouring more and more money into health care delivery. This has been accomplished through contracting with the private sector: Medicare contracts, PRO contracts, etc. In fact, about 61 cents of every dollar expended on healthcare comes from the government. As we move to a universal access system, I think that all care will be contracted out...at the least cost in bureaucratic disruption. But to do so—and to keep costs within manageable limits—efforts must be made to limit access to care, control the content of that care, and to assess the effectiveness of care (and eventually for determining priority funding as well as for assuring accountability). Initially, care will be "rationed" by setting caps. Priority decisions most likely will be left to providers. However, eventually, improved and extensive outcome data will be used to determine funding in priorities at state and national levels. Let's see how the three premises that undergird today's move to outcomes management are moving healthcare in a new direction. Those premises are: 1) quality of care is necessary care; 2) quality of care is care delivered to standard; and 3) quality of care is measurable and comparable.

Quality of care is necessary care

Suppose a surgeon amputated my leg, my recovery was unremarkable and my rehabilitation successful. Wouldn't you agree that I received quality care? Probably, but it wouldn't be "quality care" if my leg didn't need to be amputated in the first place! As the payors (government and private) began analyzing, sharing and comparing their claims data, they discovered amazing disparities in

Quality care is necessary care.

medical practice patterns: e.g., caesarean section rates varied as much as 400 percent from one geographic area to another. As a result of these discoveries, more and more payors began demanding some assurance that proposed treatments, especially hospital admissions, were necessary—and had some chance of doing any good. Thus, the demand for precertification. In the near future, precertification demands will (and in some cases already do) include precertification even for emergency admissions. Payors will pay for "holding" a patient for 23 hours and 59 minutes while laboratory and x-ray tests justify admissions decisions. However, they are unlikely to continue to pay for the practice of placing such patients in empty med/surg beds scattered throughout the institution. Rather, "holding" patients will have to be placed in monitored beds with staffing appropriate to the level of observation their condition requires. Holding areas adjacent to emergency departments seem an ideal solution.

Moreover, admissions to critical care areas will have to be "precertified" or "justified" by a screening tool—most likely the APACHE III. Otherwise the admission will not be covered.

Quality care is necessary care. And the determination and justification procedures being developed are about as unbiased a way to control access to both hospitals and high tech care as one can find. Not only can they be used to limit access, they also could be used to justify discharge...either because the patient no longer "needs" a given level of care or because the patient's situation has deteriorated to being irreversibly terminal.

Quality of care is care delivered to standard

Could anyone argue that substandard care is acceptable—or should be reimbursable? I think not...or, at least, not successfully. But how will standards be set and who will set them? Articulating medical practice guidelines and tying them to reimbursement is inevitable. Both the IOM and the AMA are deeply involved in mediating their development, and 27 medical specialty groups already have published diagnosed-based medical practice guidelines. Once physician reimbursement is tied to medical practice guidelines, compliance is all but assured. Make no mistake about it: the guidelines not only will guard against substandard practice but also strongly discourage "supra" standard practice. Thus, medical practice guidelines or "standards" can be used to control the content of medical practice, and through that, the cost of care.

Guidelines not only will guard against substandard practice but also strongly discourage "supra" standard practice.

Not only physicians but also hospitals will be held fiscally accountable for delivering "standard" care. Sharing the hospital's quality assurance track record is likely to be a prerequisite for contract negotiations in public and private sectors alike. More: hospital quality indices which compare one hospital with another will be published to help the public as well as the payor make informed choices.

Quality of care is measurable and comparable

While almost everyone—payors, regulators and professionals—agree that current performance data are inadequate, the general consensus is that the available data, however unsatisfactory, will be used. Moreover, the huge data sets which are emerging from diverse sources will be used to determine the comparative effectiveness of various clinical decisions and procedures. These in turn can and probably will largely determine funding priorities.

Quality of care is measurable and comparable. That is, it is effective. Effectiveness is determined by statistical analysis and comparison. As surely as day follows night, the development of any universal access program will shift money away from high-risk, highly invasive interventions and redirect it toward the low-risk, lower tech interventions that most people need. We are talking about opening access to at least basic care for 69 million people and improving access to "standard" care for the 60 million underinsured.

None of this will be achieved without pain. The revolution begins anew...and high-tech, highly-invasive, high-risk medical practices will be among the first casualties. The wheels are already in motion.

June 1991

HEALTH ISSUES: FROM RHETORIC TO REFORM

In his book, *You Don't Have to Be in Who's Who to Know What's What*, Sam Levenson made the following observation: "...Every mortal in the eternal, though involuntary, process of returning dust to dust sooner or later finds (or gropes) his way to another mortal called 'doctor' in the hope that the latter may conjure up some potion potent enough to dissolve the dust that time has deposited in his eyes, ears, nose, throat, arteries..." This process of keeping our life-sustaining system of pumps, valves and organs dustfree is growing increasingly expensive. Appallingly so.

One million four hundred thirty-eight thousand three hundred fifty dollars ($1,438,350) per minute. Or, if you prefer, twenty-three thousand nine hundred thirty dollars ($23,930) per second. That's what Americans spent on healthcare last year.

From witch doctors to rich doctors

"In ancient times, the witch doctor looked after the health of his tribe *gratis*," Levenson said, "in return for which he was treated like a high priest. Now that we're no longer primitive, and now that the doctor expects to get paid, he is no longer treated like a high priest but like a highway robber. The doctors' switch from free to fee earned him both a living and the chronic resentment of the people." Witness the blatant anti-physician and anti-medicine attitudes on Capitol Hill. Of course, this attitude is not improved when physicians lobby in such a way that they are perceived as self-interested and sniveling. Pennsylvania's Senator Harris Wofford won a surprise, come-from-behind victory principally because of his dramatic call for national health insurance. His healthcare message was simple: "If criminals have a right to a lawyer, working Americans have a right to a doctor." Healthcare reform—and the eventual destruction of the fee-for-service system—is *the* issue of the 90s (see Exhibit I).

EXHIBIT I

25 HEALTH ISSUES: HOW THEY FARED IN 1991, AND WHERE THEY'LL GO IN 1992

Issue	1991 Progress/Regress	Implications for 1992
Abortion	On May 23, the Supreme Court upheld the 1988 HHS regulation barring abortion counseling at family planning clinics funded under Title X of the Public Health Service Act.	Pro-choice groups will push for a Supreme Court decision before the 1992 elections. ACLU and PPF want the Court to examine a Pennsylvania law limiting abortion.
AIDS	More than 200,000 cases have been reported and more than 130,000 have died. In 1991, 45,000 new cases were reported, and 18,325 people died; costs for care will reach $10.4 billion by 1994. Opposition from medical and health groups forced the CDC to withdraw guidelines limiting the activities of HIV- infected health professionals. The new proposal limits only those HCWs who are physically or mentally impaired.	The CDC wants to expand the definition of AIDS to include those infected with HIV who have fewer than 200 CD4 cells per mm of blood. The SSA disagrees. At stake are disability benefits—especially for women and children. Look for more political fireworks over testing and/or limiting the activities of HIV positive HCWs.
Administrative costs	Healthcare prices continue to outstrip inflation in the general economy by a 2:1 margin. The health tab hit about $725 billion in 1991. Backers of national health insurance claim that reforming the U.S. systems could save $100 billion by cutting red tape. HHS secretary Sullivan disagrees, but holds a "summit" with insurers to seek solutions.	Look for political pressure to reform the health system. Currently, Bush's Advisory Council on Social Security wants the Feds to lay out $7 billion to increase access for 20 million uninsured Americans. Of the total, $3 billion will help states test prototype reform plans. The push is to cover all uninsured—and to control costs. This plan does neither. No one is satisfied.
Aging	The National Institute on Aging launched a $2.2 million study to determine the benefits of nursing home special care units for Alzheimer's disease and senile dementia. The IOM called for a 33% increase in funding for research on aging.	The White House set a post election 1993 date for a Conference on Aging.
Assisted suicide	Derek Humphry's book, Final Exit—a primer on "how to kill yourself"—hit the best-seller list. Dr. Jack Kevorkian ended the year by helping two women, neither of whom was terminally ill, to kill themselves. Nonetheless, Washington voters soundly rejected a proposal to legalize euthanasia.	The push to legalize mercy killing will continue—with the Hemlock Society leading the way. California, Colorado, and Oregon will have initiatives introduced into their state legislation. The public's fear of being forced to undergo futile treatment adds fuel to this drive. The Patient Self-Determination Act, if properly and humanely implemented, could help defuse this issue.
Clinical labs	Regulations implementing 1988 legislation were finally published.	Implementations of regulations will be slowed by the difficulties encountered in dealing with thousands of small laboratories.
Drugs	Drug industry increases in prices angered Congress. The FDA announced plans to speed up review of new drugs. The House passed a bill that would give the FDA more authority to penalize generic drug makers who engage in fraudulent acts.	Look for legislation that will strip drug makers of tax breaks if price hikes don't abate—or even roll back.

(continued)

231

EXHIBIT I

25 HEALTH ISSUES: HOW THEY FARED IN 1991 *(continued)*

Issue	1991 Progress/Regress	Implications for 1992
Emergency care	Trauma care is getting worse. A 40-state survey of 240 teaching hospitals indicates that, in nearly half of them, emergency patients wait an average of 10 hours for a bed.	Prohibitive regulations will lead even more hospitals to drop their status as trauma centers.
Geographic reclassifications	Almost 1,000 rural and suburban hospitals were reclassified into higher Medicare reimbursement categories—a move which cost other facilities about $450 million.	Another 1,350 facilities will seek reclassification in 1992. Despite AHA opposition, about half will succeed.
HMOs	HCFA enforced the Medicare HMO program. The GAO's study finds certain HMOs guilty of abuse, particularly Humana's Florida Plan.	Look for stricter enforcement—and the implementation of electronic billing before the year 2000.
HCWs	The Labor Department finally published regulations to protect HCWs from bloodborne infections, especially HIV and hepatitis B.	None
Infectious disease	Massive increase in antibiotic-resistant tuberculosis raises concerns. Immunization rates among low-income, minority pre-schoolers are as low as 50%. The Bush Administration launched a campaign to increase access to immunization.	Emphasis on personal responsibility, healthy lifestyle, and immunization will continue.
Long-term care	HCFA approved Connecticut's plans to mix private long-term care insurance with Medicaid coverage. HCFA and California worked to implement 1987 nursing home reform law that the state says is too cumbersome.	Indiana and other states will follow Connecticut's lead. With the growth in the number of seniors, the push for nursing home reform will continue.
Medicaid	Hospitals were reimbursed an average of 78 cents on the dollar (down from 90 cents in 1985) for Medicaid patients—and the PPRC says it would cost $2.4 billion a year for Medicaid to match Medicare rates.	Look for Congress to move to match rates as a compromise as politicians continue to argue over health reform.
Medical devices	Providers began reporting to the FDA incidents suggesting that medical devices caused or contributed to patients' injuries or illnesses. Insurers and managed care groups offer to give $1 million to the government to double the number of annual reviews of new technology.	Regulators and lawmakers will seek ways to police device makers who bilk Medicare recipients. Despite device makers' attempts to stall efforts to increase the new technology reviews, the plan will get through in 1992.
Medigap	HHS designated 15 states where Medicare beneficiaries can enroll on PPOs to buy cheaper Medigap coverage.	None

EXHIBIT I

25 HEALTH ISSUES: HOW THEY FARED IN 1991 *(continued)*

Issue	1991 Progress/Regress	Implications for 1992
Military health care	Congress expanded the Pentagon's experiment with managed care from 2 to 6 states and extended California and Hawaii's managed care program to February 1, 1994.	None
Ophthalmology	HCFA proposed to bundle Medicare payments for cataract surgery.	Ophthalmologists will seek a legislative block, but will fail on this one.
Organ transplants	Researchers report that blacks are at four times the risk of kidney failure as are whites—and less likely to get a transplant. The low priority given to transplantation in rationing schemes (e.g. Oregon) raises consumer concerns.	Problems of distribution, social justice, and costs will continue to plague transplant programs.
Physician referrals	Regulations aim to curb the practice of physicians referring to facilities in which they have an interest. At the year's end, AMA proposed further limits. However, HHS created 11 exceptions to Medicare/Medicaid anti-kickback laws.	Physician/hospital joint ventures are dead or dying. Consumer demands for social accountability will limit the profitability of medical for-profit ventures.
Patient dumping	HHS won an important anti-dumping case in Texas where Michael Burdett, MD, was fined $20,000 for violating federal anti-dumping laws.	Look for HHS to crack down on patient dumping in 1992.
Rationing	Oregon's rationing scheme, which "prioritizes" medical services to the poor, raises debate. Politics and posturing interfere with the federal waiver necessary to begin implementation.	The Oregon federal waiver of Medicaid rules probably will be granted by July of 1992.
Research	Following allegations of overcharging, the government limited how much it will pay for universities' indirect medical research costs.	An HHS task force will make recommendations for a crackdown on indirect research costs.
Unions	The Supreme Court upheld a 1989 NLRB ruling allowing 8 separate collective bargaining units in acute care hospitals.	Look for an increase in union activities, especially among RNs.
Women's health	NIH launched a 10-year, $500 million study of the effects of diet, hormone use, and smoking on diseases that affect women.	Look for more interest in the health of women.

...lead to debate and action

The healthcare cost juggernaut reels forward, out of control despite a weak economy and growing public discontent. While the Administration studies the problem to death and politicians prattle about it, the system decays around them (see Exhibit). Business claims that healthcare costs are eating up 49 percent of corporate profits. Unions complain about a rollback in health benefits. Thirty-eight million Americans are medically indigent.

And physician income rose yet again in 1991. While there was little progress on access to care in 1991, the groundwork has been laid for healthy debate in 1992 which will lead to real action in 1993. One of the targets will be the way—and the amount—physicians are paid. 1991 saw considerable action in this regard: a new national fee schedule for physicians was implemented and a new Medicare capital payment system was put in place for hospitals (see Exhibit for further issues). Hospital costs and physician payment will be at the center of the health reform debate in 1992.

Non-physician providers (especially nurses) will have the best chance in decades to make an impact. To do so, nurses need a working knowledge of major health issues—and workable, incremental approaches to their resolution. The approaches must include close, collaborative relationships with physicians. When nurses are seen as lobbying only for their own self-interest, they lose their effectiveness. The cost crisis in healthcare was not caused solely by physicians, but it *cannot* be solved without them. A healthy and mutual respect, augmented by a genuine knowledge of one another's abilities, must underlie a joint determination to genuinely reform the healthcare system.

I said earlier that it can't be done without doctors. I'll say now, it can't be done without nurses either. We must work together to find a potion potent enough to revivify a system crumbling from within. No more self-interest or sniveling. Just do it.

February 1992

Signs of Things to Come

A tradition of Haverford College centers around the administration of its famous President, Dr. William Wistar Comfort. When Dr. Comfort had a beautiful sign proclaiming the college's name placed at the campus entrance, an enterprising group of seniors stole the sign and hid it.

The sign was missing for many days during which the President instituted a search, found the sign, removed it, and hid it in his own quarters. He then announced to the student body that, although a joke was a joke, unless the sign was returned by Saturday night, he would revoke all privileges of the senior class indefinitely.

Accordingly, an extremely glum and down-in-the-mouth group of seniors assembled in chapel the Sunday morning after the deadline. Dr. Comfort stepped into the pulpit, surveyed the faces before him and opened the great Bible. Solemnly, he intoned the day's text: "A wicked and adulterous generation seeketh for a sign and there shall be none given unto them."

> **Harbingers of the future: they are there—and we could make a better future sooner if we would heed them.**

Signs, portents, harbingers of the future: we all claim to seek but rarely find them. So we hunker down against the winds of change and stumble along as best we can without them. Although somewhat obscured by the exigencies of daily problems, they *are* there—and we could make a better future sooner if we *would* heed them.

To uncover the signs of the future, the *Healthcare Forum Leadership Center* queried over 2500 healthcare opinion leaders (400 responded), interviewed management experts, conducted a literature search, and sponsored a series of focus groups.

Facts calling for change

Their study presented the participants with three future scenarios based upon some commonly held facts and perceptions about the state of American healthcare.

The cost of maintaining our current system will reach 2 trillion dollars per year—fully 17 percent of the GNP—by the year 2000.

- In a recent Harris poll, 90 percent of Americans said that the U.S. healthcare system needs fundamental restructuring.
- Health expenditures reached $738 billion in 1991—almost 13 percent of the GNP.
- Costs for health benefits for employees are rising nearly 12 percent per year—eating up 48 percent of corporate profits and forcing small companies to drop their health insurance benefits.
- At least 35 million citizens lack health coverage—and almost 75 percent of them are working Americans and their children.
- We aren't even getting value for the social dollars we spend—U.S. health status ranks poorly relative to other post-industrial societies as indicated by measures such as infant mortality, average life expectancy and morbidity.

Five trends shaping the future

There are also other matters to consider: those economic, technological and sociological more-or-less "megatrends" that will mold the facts into new sets of statistics.

- The incidence and prevalence of chronic, long-term lifestyle related diseases—in an aging society: Today we have about 30 million people over the age of 65, roughly 10 percent of whom are over the age of 85. By 2015 we will have almost 60 million people over the age of 65 and *16 million over the age of 85.*

- The costs of maintaining our current system, while fewer and fewer Americans gain access to it: Those costs will reach $2 trillion dollars per year—fully 17 percent of the GNP—by the year 2000.
- Advancing technologies in a shrinking delivery system: Highly invasive and expensive procedures focus resources on the few—some say, at the expense of the many.
- Rising payor participation in determining resource allocation: Purchasers have more power than ever before. Their power is posed in opposition to medicine's autonomy in many instances—and this "Cold War" is threatening to break out into guerrilla warfare. Non-combatants (patients and families) are the victims.
- Failure of competition as an effective strategy in the health sector of the economy: Competition has produced less access to lower quality services at a horrendous waste of resources.

Three future scenarios

Keeping these elements of the plot in mind, let us consider the three scenarios *Healthcare Forum* placed before their study participants.

1. Continued Growth/High Tech: The U.S. health system expands with the economy, reaching 17 percent of the GNP by 2001. High-tech proliferates, providing cures and extending lives, but at high cost. *Healthcare reform did not occur.* Managed care grows but patchwork coverage persists. Medical indigency increases along with unequal access.

> **The only reason for predicting the future is to prepare for its coming or to change its direction and pace.**

2. Hard Times/Government Leadership: A persistent recession leads to the political necessity to develop a universal access system. The result is a frugal, Canadian-like national health insurance system with significant rationing of services (especially highly technical ones) based on cost/benefit and outcomes research. Heroic life-

237

EXHIBIT I

1. STRATEGIC LEADERSHIP ORIENTATION

Conventional Practice		Transformational Practices
Business planning	→	Shared vision
Minimizing risks	→	Mastering change
Repairing body parts	→	Redefining healthcare
Maximizing short-term profits	→	Serving the public/community
Linear learning	→	Systems thinking
Business boundaries	→	Global approach
Homogeneous culture	→	Managing diverse workforces

2. MANAGING PEOPLE AND PROJECTS

Conventional Tactics		Transformational Tactics
Protecting self-interest	→	CQI
Individual learning	→	Team learning
Hierarchical management	→	Lateral cross-functional structure
Incentive-based compensation	→	Fostering enrollment
Using marketing techniques	→	Promoting customer relations

3. HARNESSING TECHNOLOGY

Conventional Use		Transformational Use
Invasive diagnostics and therapeutics	→	Non-invasive diagnostics and therapeutics
Capital budgeting for technology	→	Strategic technology assessment
Minimizing existing technology	→	Building information technology
Employing technology specialists	→	Diffusing technology through user-friendly applications

saving measures decline and researchers adopt a more frugal approach to innovation. Healthcare's percentage of the GNP shrinks to 11 percent by 2001.

3. New Civilization: Dramatic changes in science, technology, society and government hasten healthcare change. Care broadens its focus from the person to the community and the environment. National health reform favors managed care through a government/business sector partnership with discretion at the community level. That partnership provides basic coverage for all with an emphasis on the continuum of care, health promotion and "social

HMOs." High tech and alternative therapies are common. Healthcare consumes 12 percent of the GNP in 2001.

What we say/what we do

Nearly nine out of ten (87%) of the opinion leaders *preferred* the "New Civilization" scenario. Nevertheless, they thought that, of the three, this one was least likely to transpire. By a slight margin the leaders thought that the "Hard Times/Government Leadership" was more likely to take place than the "Continued Growth/High Tech" scenario.

The only reason for predicting the future is to prepare for its coming or to change its direction and pace. *Healthcare Forum Leadership Center's* survey reports that leaders do see significant gaps between their current practices and those the future requires. Exhibit I charts the contrasts.

Whether this generation can be ranked among the "wicked and adulterous" ones, I leave to you. Certainly, it has been greedy. Now, mightily dismayed, this generation "seeketh for a sign"...and more than one has been given unto it.

In the end, the *future* will become the *present* people want. Really want. Want badly enough to change their minds and habits for. Want badly enough to work and save for. Want badly enough to pay the price.

July 1992

HEALTH REFORM: EVERYBODY PLAYS AND EVERYBODY PAYS

Historian John Bach McMaster tells this story about Abraham Lincoln. Taken as a young boy to a White House reception, McMaster watched the guests line up and be escorted under the watchful eyes of the ushers, past the Civil War President. No one was allowed close enough to shake his hand or to speak to him. One disappointed old-timer, having come a long way just for this occasion, waved his hat and shouted from the end of the line: "Mr President, I'm from up in New York state where we believe that God Almighty and Abraham Lincoln are going to save this country." Smiling, the President returned the wave and jovially called out to him, "My friend, you're half right."

The federal deficit

Heaven knows that we need someone to be half right if we are going to calm down this nation's current domestic crisis. Carol Cox Wait, president of the nonprofit Committee for a Responsible Federal Budget, minces no words: "The budget debate has become a healthcare debate..." And as Senator Bob Kerry (D-NE) declared on the Senate floor in June, "Healthcare entitlements are driving the [federal budget] deficit." Members of Congress, policy gurus and budget watchers agreeing.

Certainly, there's no denying the figures. Federal per capita outlays for healthcare alone grew 54 percent in the 1980s. Thank God we were being frugal! Even if entitlements are not expanded, the 1990s look no better. Medicare and Medicaid will constitute 85 percent of the growth in entitlement spending between 1993 and 1997.

About two-thirds of the federal budget ($978 billion in 1992) goes to mandatory spending programs: $300 billion goes to Social Security, $210 billion is earmarked for Medicare and Medicaid, and it takes $214 billion just to pay the *interest* on the deficit. To top this, spending rises automatically to cover not only inflation and increasing numbers of beneficiaries, but also rising indebtedness: we added another $350 billion to push the federal deficit to about $3 trillion last year alone. (The other one-third of the federal budget goes for discretionary programs, e.g., $270 billion for the military and $15 billion for the U.S. Public Health Service.)

> **The fear of becoming indigent from paying medical bills is the heart of the matter.**

Despite DRGs, freezes on physician fees and lame attempts at "economic incentives," Medicare spending increased some 12.2 percent every year during the 1980s. Medicaid's average annual increase was "only" 11.4 percent—but in 1991 Medicaid had risen by 18.8 percent, and a 27.8 percent increase is predicted for 1992. To staunch this flow, Capitol Hill and White House alike contemplate—albeit from different perspectives—legislation which would change the rules of *eligibility* and/or *reimbursement*.

Which do you think it ought to be?

Of politics and penury

To understand the politics involved, you must locate healthcare reform in the center of this truly grim economic picture.

QUESTION: With the nation staggering under a $3 trillion debt and with Medicare and Medicaid costs spiraling out of control, why would any politician in his right mind *even consider* proposing another healthcare entitlement program?

ANSWER: To get elected...or re-elected.

For over a decade, most Americans have watched their own health benefits shrink or even disappear while, at the same time, revenues from the taxes and premiums they worked and paid for are drained away to deliver healthcare to strangers.

Both parties agree on the approximate number of "uninsureds" in this country: about 35.5 million. Neither party is talking about the fact that the vast majority (about 80%) of the uninsured are working, tax-paying Americans and their dependents. Moreover, high insurance premiums are compelling business and industry to abandon health benefit programs for their employees. A George Washington University study released in May 1992 indicates that as many as 55 million Americans will be among the uninsured by December of this year.

Some have defined the problem in terms of access to care. That is not the problem. Medical indigents—or more precisely the fear of becoming indigent from paying medical bills—is the heart of the matter. Many, if not most, uninsureds can get at least some degree of care in emergency rooms and clinics if nowhere else. They just can't *pay* for it without Draconian sacrifice or, sometimes, complete financial disaster. One serious injury, one bout with cancer, one major surgery, and their children's college education, their savings, and their basic security are gone. All they've worked for all their lives—and then some—slides into someone else's pocket: doctor, hospital, DME company, pharmacists, laboratory, rehab.

And they are afraid.

Even insured workers—with good cause—fear that they, too, will lose their benefits "the way things are going." This fear, fueled by a loss of job security in a persistent recession, drives the demand for health reform: a formidable force indeed.

In the tinder box

Add to this fear the frustration of those denied insurance themselves who realize they are paying for what appears to be unlimited healthcare for others. Case in point: Oregon was denied a Medicaid waiver last summer.

In 1989, Oregon's legislature voted to expand the state's Medicaid program and its coverage to 120,000 Oregonians at or below the poverty level. Moreover, fully implemented, the program would extend insurance coverage to 300,000 of Oregon's uninsured state residents whose incomes are above the poverty line. To pay for this, Oregon developed a complex plan to rate and rank the 700 medical procedures covered by Medicaid. Then lawmakers drew a line below which the state would no longer cover a service.

Let's get the record straight. In 1987—two years *before* this legislation passed—Oregon ended coverage of organ transplants, except kidney and cornea. This freed money to add 3,000 women and children to the Medicaid rolls. Federal law does not require state Medicaid programs to provide transplants to anyone—and most do not.

In 1989, Oregon's state legislature prioritized the list of covered medical services to fund *all* services "essential to basic health-care," and 82 percent of services regarded as "very important," as well as seven percent of conditions categorized as "valuable to individuals but of minimal gain or high cost."

While the state wanted to expand coverage to preventive care, it would have excluded coverage for: viral hepatitis, chronic bronchitis, viral pneumonia, liver transplants for alcoholics with cirrhosis of the liver, medical therapy for terminal AIDS patients and cancer patients, and "excessive" treatment for premature infants under 500 grams.

The Bush Administration rejected the Oregon waiver—and thus put an end to Oregon's universal access experiment—because it claimed the Oregon plan violated the 1990 *Americans with Disabilities Act*. The Administration cited as two specific examples for discrimination: eliminating coverage for liver transplants for alcoholics with cirrhosis and eliminating coverage for "excessive therapy" for premature infants whose birth weight is under 500 grams (and whose chances of survival are very slight indeed).

Oregon officials say that they based their rankings on medical effectiveness, not on "stereo-typical assumptions" about the value of life. Mark Gibson, chief of staff to Senator John Kitzhaber, MD, president of Oregon's Senate and author of the plan, concluded, "If you carry their argument to the fullest extent, [the Bush administration] is saying you can't deny futile care."

So, the federal government risks the health and welfare of 420,000 Oregonians to pay for *futile care* for a very few.

And the frustration builds into anger which, united with fear, fills the tinder box. All we need now is the match.

Healthcare reform

Apparently the 33 million elderly and disabled people covered by Medicare, along with the citizens who *do* meet state eligibility requirements for Medicaid, have almost unlimited coverage if they are handicapped. Astounding yearly increases demonstrate the extent of that coverage. Furthermore, simple arithmetic seems to indicate that adding 35 million uninsured would sky-rocket costs which in turn will burn up any efforts to reduce the federal deficit.

One thing is for sure, economists agree that *nothing* will keep healthcare expenditures from reaching $1.2 trillion a year by 1995. At 15 percent of the GNP, the American consuming public will explode: they're darn close to it now. And everyone will pay.

What is likely to happen? The government will:

And the frustration builds into anger which, united with fear, fills the tinder box. All we need now is the match.

- Cap physician fees and hospital costs stringently
- Limit Medicare benefits to the elderly whose incomes are above $50,000/year
- Cap or eliminate the tax exclusion people get for employer-provided health insurance
- Adopt some of the "pay or play" approaches which require employers to provide insurance or pay a tax
- Subsidize insurance for workers over age 60 and other high-cost patients

A proposal from paradise

Hawaii's health plan covers 98 percent of its population. Yet, its per capita costs are the lowest in the nation. In 1991, the amount of the Gross State Product Hawaii residents spent on healthcare was below nine percent (the national figure was 14+%).

Hawaii's Director of Health, John C. Lewin, MD, proposes the following 10 steps for Federal health reform:

1. "Congress must establish a standard benefit package for all Americans...

2. "A federal employer-mandate, similar to the ERISA exempted "everybody plays" model Hawaii uses, should be the foundation of private coverage [employers, employees and the state *all* pay]...

3. "Insurers should be required to offer open enrollment and true community ratings; and exclusions, restrictions and waiting periods would be eliminated...co-payments and deductions would be held within caps...

4. "Each year the government would establish a threshold of how much of insurance premiums would be tax-deductible...based on the most cost-effective and quality premiums for employed people in each state...

5. "The federal funding to states for Medicaid, disproportionate share hospital subsidies, community health center funding, certain categorical public health funds, and any other federal healthcare funding to states, must be available in flexible blocks or grants to enable states to guarantee coverage to the unemployed, the poor, and other special populations not covered by private insurance through employment or retirement...

6. "The federal government would need to establish standardized and simple claim forms for use by all insurers, public and private...

7. "The so-called proprietary information related to insurance, provider, hospital and other costs of healthcare must be made public...to create a cost-competitive healthcare market place in America...

8. "A small amount of funds must be set aside at the federal and state level to develop and staff high-level appointed commissions charged to monitor and study healthcare costs, consumer and provider behavior and satisfaction, and health status and outcomes with respect to costs of care...

9. "The federal government needs to establish a national policy and cost containment strategy in [regard to tort reform].

10. "...We must devote resources and attention to public health, health promotion and education, and prevention through a congressionally-legislated additional set-aside of at least three percent of all federal healthcare expenditures..."

Universal access to health insurance coverage is possible. We can cut costs. We can improve the public's health. And we can even begin to reduce the federal deficit. But only if all players are as willing to "ante up" as they are to "take the pot."

Not only is that the only way that health reform makes sense...it's the only way health reform is possible. *Everybody plays and everybody pays.*

November 1992

THRIVING ON CHAOS

Many health professionals are finding that, soulwise, these are trying times. It seems that the United States has elected its first health-reform-wonk (wind him up and he talks healthcare) as president. To be the subject of reform—not to mention being portrayed as hard-hearted despoilers of the Medicare system—strikes most of us as darned hard cheese. Duty requires the earnest nurse to spend most of her/his time on the *qui vive* for medical excesses, be in a state of profound depression over the advance of the medical-industrial complex, and to be down in the dumps over the incredible naivete of administrators who think they can increase productivity yet again.

Colleagues, fear not, neither let your hearts be weary. Rejoice, I bring you glad tidings. I have spent the whole of my professional career in a climate at least as chaotic as that being created by Bill Clinton and his band of merry reformers; and I assure you, *this* not only can be endured, it can be

Things are not getting worse; things have always been this bad.

enjoyed. Actually, you have two other choices: cry or throw up. Neither of these latter two is good for your health, so I recommend laughter. All you need in order to laugh about health reform is a strong stomach. A tempered steel tummy.

You have to ignore a lot of stuff in order to laugh about health reform—things like being "restructured" out of your job and such—but we can toughen up our stomachs by taking it a day at a time.

Here are three perfectly good reasons to keep laughing during health reform:

• Things are not getting worse; things have always been this bad. Few things are as consoling as the long perspective of history. It will perk you up no end to go back and read the works of retired leaders of the healthcare industry. You will learn that things back then were terrible too, and what's more, they were always getting worse. This is most inspiring.

-Dateline: 1968. The nation is undergoing health reform. Medicare and Medicaid begin implementation. The American Medical Association predicts that government interference will lead to socialism. These changes turned the world of hospitals and healthcare upside down.

-Dateline: 1982. The nation is undergoing reform again. Congress passed DRG legislation. Hospitals become competitive corporations. Physicians et al. become entrepreneurs. The American Medical Association claims that the whole system is going to hell in a handbasket and we'll be socialized before we know it. These changes turned the world of hospitals and healthcare upside down.

-Dateline: 1993. The nation is undergoing health reform yet again. The Clinton Administration is pushing for "managed competition" and "global budgets" to control health costs. The American Medical Association draws a "line in the sand" over global budgets, seeks federal antitrust relief to let physicians negotiate rates with groups, and wants change in ERISA (the Employee Retirement Income Security Act) so that self-insured benefit plans would have to negotiate with physicians. Otherwise, the American Medical Association warns, healthcare will be rationed and the system inevitably will slide into socialism. These changes turn the world of hospitals and healthcare upside down.

> **Let us give thanks for the time "managed competition" may buy us—while we still have time.**

Get the point?

- Things could be worse. The fact that they probably will get worse is no excuse for tossing away this golden opportunity to rejoice in the relative delightfulness of our current situation. Is there anything to cheer us in the realization that competition in healthcare is now to be "managed," which in turn somehow will lead to universal access? Yes. Writing in the *Futurist* magazine (26:2), Weiner predicted that the "burgeoning health insurance crisis will lead to 'health wars' in which activists for one disease (such as breast cancer) will challenge the emphasis put on another (such as AIDS)." Let us give thanks for the time "managed competition" may buy us—while we still have time.

> **...that awful tendency nurses have to bleed from the heart over victims of cruelty and injustice.**

- There is always the off-chance that adversity will improve our character. Since we are all the spiritual children of the Puritans (though mostly "fallen-away"), we secretly believe that suffering is good for the soul. Constant chaos sort of keeps you on your toes. I'm taking this opportunity to catch up on my non-health related reading which, so far has added to my anxiety. Consider the following predictions:

1. the number of people working two jobs will increase and worker wakefulness will be an issue of growing concern...

2. members of the baby-bust generation now entering the workforce tend to have a terrible work ethic and don't bow to any authority...

3. managers are starting to keep "electronic dossiers" on their employees' electronic mail and fax messages...

Oh well, I can always console myself with one further prediction: "Future offices may have rooms for karate, meditation, communal cooking, or even sexual activity breaks..." (*The Futurist* 26:6).

I'm also working hard to counter that awful tendency nurses have to bleed from the heart over victims of cruelty and injustice. One of my New Year's resolutions is *not* to feel sorry for the physician groups who have purchased MRIs or built their own little private "intensive care hospitals" (guaranteed 50 percent return on investment the first year—after that, it's all gravy). I've hardly ever heard of anything so awfully unfair as the legislation making it illegal for physicians to refer Medicare patients to facilities in which the physician has a financial interest. And now the American Medical Association has gone on record discouraging such self-referral (research shows that physicians who own MRIs order 40 percent more MRIs than those who don't, etc.). Gosh, it's a good thing I have a will of iron or I'd be hard put to suppress those little twinges of sympathy.

Watching the reactions to the Clinton Administration's appointees should keep political satirists like Mark Russell full of glee for the rest of the year, too. From the time Clinton selected Donna Shalala to head HHS, and former CBO director Alice Rivlin coupled with Leon Panetta, House Budget Committee Chairman, to head the Office of Management and Budget, the nay-sayers have been swallowing their tongues, most notably the Health Insurance Association of America and the American Medical Association. Managed care, global budgets, DRGs, health insurance reform, managed competition. This is great stuff, a barrel of laughs.

And underneath it all is a serious interest and a steely will. The President meant what he said during his campaign. There will be health reform. And it will be chaotic. And, like Tom Peters says, we can thrive on it. It's all a matter of perspective.

February 1993

HEALTH REFORM: LOOKING THE SNAKE IN THE EYE

Everywhere I go today, people are talking about health reform. And they are all nervous. About different things. Physicians because they are afraid their incomes will be cut and their practices controlled. Administrators because they fear reduced revenues and more regulations. Suppliers because they fear price caps or even cuts. Nurse administrators because they fear budget cuts and reduced staffing...

During any period of waiting, anxiety—fueled by fear—rises. Sometimes this leads to frenzied activity and sometimes to paralysis. Both can be fatal.

The Navaho Indians describe fear as a rattlesnake, about six feet long and as thick as a man's wrist. Avoid it and the snake grows larger and comes closer, rearing its head and baring its fangs as it gets ready to strike. If you run, it will bite you, but if you look the snake in the eye unblinkingly, it sees its own reflection, gets scared and slithers away.

Before we do anything else, let's look this snake in the eye: what's to be afraid of in the health reform proposals we've heard to date?

More money, not less

Current estimates indicate that (depending on how much we reform the system) anywhere from 30 to 150 billion *more* dollars a year will be spent on health care *if* we reform the system.

According to the latest estimates, Americans spent about 900 billion dollars on healthcare in 1992. Given healthcare's average yearly rate of inflation of 12.5 percent over the last decade, that means we will spend about one trillion one hundred and twenty five billion dollars on health and illness care in 1993. Given these kinds of figures, I think the healthcare system probably could absorb another 30 or even 150 billion dollars without too much strain. Particularly if we are to provide services for more people. A lot more people.

More people, not fewer

Both Republicans and Democrats agree: at least 38 million people have no insurance coverage, and about one hundred million people are underinsured. That is, their insurance will not cover the costs of treatment for common diseases (e.g., cancer, heart disease, etc.). Improving the basic package of care available to the latter and providing access to insurance coverage for the former is part and parcel of any health reform proposal. While opening services for 38 million people presents interesting logistical problems, they are not insurmountable. *No one is talking about shrinking the healthcare systems.*

> **About 1,000 hospitals will close their doors by the end of the decade.**

Everyone is talking about expanding it. And improving it. The government wants the healthcare system to provide services for more people and they are going to provide more money. Sounds like boom times to me.

Breaking old habits

In ancient Mesopotamia, legend has it that there was a village made famous by artisans who produced exquisite vases and urns. Some of them were as high as a man's shoulder, and all of them were uncommonly strong, unique and beautiful. The reason: after each piece was fired, the artist broke it—and then painstakingly put it back together with gold filigree.

I think that just about everyone in or associated with the healthcare system is afraid of being broken. They relate more to Humpty-Dumpty than the Mesopotamian urn.

Expert prognosticators claim that about 1,000 hospitals will close their doors by the end of the decade. They are probably right. But they were saying the same thing before the current furor over reform. Why? Because competition is bankrupting them. Under health reform, those one thousand hospitals will switch function rather than cease to function. They're likely to be converted to satellite urgi-centers and surgi-centers. Some may even convert their inpatient beds to skilled nursing or rehabilitation beds. A change, but hardly a matter for despair. The Honorable Elaine McCoy, Canada's Minister of Labour, had this to say about experts (*Interview*, August 1990): "Experts are often too full of facts about what didn't work in the past to make the leap to the future. What the experts can never tell us is "where to go from here"...Most important political choices have to do with human values, not just expert information, and have to be made with heart."

Going with the flow

Breaking old patterns, reforming new ones to meet new demands is hardly a prescription for disaster. It is the beginning of a new venture. Practitioners of Aikido, a form of martial arts, are taught *not* to resist an attacking force. They learn to blend their power with the attacker's force and thus combine energies for their own advantage. To resist force is to court injury and defeat. It is not effortless, it takes intense planning, training, and the ability to master one's natural instincts.

> "We are willing to sacrifice, but we want to make sure that we don't give up any more than anyone else."

Right now, everyone seems to be in a holding pattern; waiting to see what's going to happen. And waiting adds to the anxiety. Lobbyists are gearing up to resist reform—or failing that, to protect their special interest group from anything that even looks like it could hurt them.

At the recent AONE convention, a "town hall" type meeting was held. Nursing administrators from throughout the country were given an opportunity to question key figures in the health reform debate: the President of the A.H.A., the Chief Lobbyist for the Consumer's Union, the head of the American Academy of Family Practitioners, the chief lobbyist for the health insurers and so forth. I was able to ask one question. It was: "How far do you think the stakeholders you represent are willing to compromise in order to achieve health reform?" Each answered in effect, "We are willing to sacrifice, but we want to make sure that we don't give up any more than anyone else." They are playing not to lose. This is something like going into a marriage with the intention of giving no more than you get. I wouldn't bet a quarter on their chances of succeeding.

Cutting and chopping doesn't work

Meanwhile, on the home front, hospitals are playing "not to lose," too. Their strategies: call a lot of meetings, cut everything, send lots of memos and copies to everyone, establish committees, eliminate services. Playing not to lose is a no-win game.

> The "cut and chop" mentality lowers morale, sows seeds of discontent among staff, and forces a kind of dreary conformity that stifles creativity, innovation and motivation as well.

In sports, the factor that separates the peak performers from the rest of the pack usually is not their level of skill. It is how they think and act under pressure. They are bold and decisive: they don't play it safe. They play to win.

While it may seem reasonable to get "leaner and meaner" in uncertain times, you pay a high price for it. The "cut and chop" mentality lowers morale, sows seeds of discontent among staff, and forces a kind of dreary conformity that stifles creativity, innovation and motivation as well. The April 9, 1990 edition of *Fortune* magazine (p.40) reported that despite (or because of?) the layoffs and increased automation, U.S. productivity "crept up by a scant 1.2 percent a year on average in the eighties...That's virtually no improvement from the seventies...More than half the 1,468 restructured companies surveyed by the Society for Human Resources Management reported that employee productivity either stayed the same or deteriorated after layoffs...Seventy-four percent of managers at downsized companies said their workers had lower morale and distrusted management...nervousness and gloom cost money...Bell and Howell determined that at least 11 percent of profits—millions of dollars—were lost to the 'lean and mean blues' of their *retained* employees." In short, layoffs get you nowhere.

Playing to win

Cutting services never increases business. It cannot. And cutting staff doesn't increase efficiency. What does? High morale. New projects. Fair treatment. Clear goals. Feeling valued. Knowing your work is important. Taking charge. Coming alive again.

Winners 'scope out the direction of change and throw their weight into it. They aren't cynical and they don't sit around telling "Hillary jokes" while they cut staff. The winners are far too busy forming strategic partnerships, building service networks, cross-training personnel, redeploying resources and developing flexible alternative plans for contingency situations. Their values and their vision are clear.

While the losers "play it safe" on the advice of experts, the winners are already out there changing the system. They've looked the snake in the eye and channeled their energy into action. And when they put the system back together again, they will—like the Mesopotamian urns—be stronger than ever. The best healthcare system in the world.

July 1993

HEALTH REFORM PROPOSALS: WHICH IS THE FAIREST OF THEM ALL?

There are times in one's life when one must go over something again and again, even though one is thoroughly sick of it. For me, Health Reform is a case in point. I know it is important—more than that, mind-bogglingly critical. I know it will have unprecedented impact on healthcare institutions, nursing roles, and patients and families. I even know that it will affect me personally as a nurse, as a parent of uninsured young adults and as a taxpayer. Nonetheless, I have read about it, studied it, tracked it and explored the politics of it for so long that—now that it's here—I'm just plain tired of it. With this caveat in mind, and with the reader cautioned to continue at his/her own risk, I can now honestly and ethically proceed to comment.

At rock bottom, the Clinton plan would set up managed competition in which networks called *Regional Health Alliances* would compete to sell *comprehensive* health insurance packages that meet governmental requirements. All employers would be required to provide insurance coverage for employees: employers would have to pick up 80 percent of the cost, employees 20 percent. There would be a cap on how much any employer would have to pay per employee. Eventually, Medicaid would be folded into the Health Alliances and care for the poor, as well as the unemployed, would be subsidized by the government. Every American would carry a national health identity card which guarantees access to care. No card, no care.

Now that the plan has been released, the battle has been engaged in earnest and fur is flying in all directions. Everyone's lobbyists are meeting and greeting, wheeling and dealing: who do you know and what do you want? We'll get it for you for a price. Whatever your opinion, hire a fancy (and expensive) P.R. firm to influence the public and lawmakers alike: they guarantee results.

Demagoguery, grandstanding and money-grubbing are at their worst, but it is un-American not to participate.

Amidst all this hoopla, claims and counter-claims fly, politicians position themselves for re-election—and a great deal of misinformation is spread about every aspect of health reform. Words and phrases like "caps," "price controls," "limits on care," "free choice" are used to propagandize rather than inform the public. Meanwhile, little is said about the expanded access and increased range of services that would be made available to most Americans. And what is said is often placed in the context of taking *it* away from some other group—usually Medicare, which actually is untouched by the Clinton Health Reform Proposal, or Medicaid, which actually is incorporated *into* the proposal. Some of the claims are so downright foolish that it's hard to believe that anyone could believe them, but they do.

> **Demagoguery, grandstanding and money-grubbing are at their worst, but it is un-American not to participate.**

First and foremost, I am astounded that anyone with a shred of common sense and even a modicum of integrity can say that we cannot afford universal access. For crying out loud, even tiny Liechtenstein can afford it! We, the people, may decide we don't want to pay for it, but to claim that we can't pay for it is so transparently false that it's painfully embarrassing. If we have other more important priorities—say, subsidizing tobacco farmers or physicians' incomes—then let's just say so.

Another thing that is irritating enough to make bile rise in one's throat is the incessant carping, nitpicking and complaining of avaricious, self-centered, "special' interest groups:

• Hiding behind the specious right to choose their own providers—a right created primarily by well-heeled public relations firms hired to do just that—consumer groups fight any governmental "interference" with their choice. No matter that most

Americans today have darn little choice of providers. No matter that hardly any Americans would have the slightest idea which specialist to choose if they ever needed one. No matter that less than half of all Americans even have a primary physician. No matter that a growing number of Americans have no choices whatsoever today. The "pro-choicers" (my apologies to the abortion movement) fight because, under the Administration's proposed reforms, consumers would only have a choice among three plans: an HMO, a PPO, or a fee-for-service indemnity plan. Ironically, this is presented to the public as a limit on their for-all-practical-purposes-today-nonexistent-choices.

• Institutional providers which fight any meaningful rate controls—despite the fact that hospital margins are higher now than at anytime in recorded history. According to PROpac, rate controls are one of only two cost control measures that really work. Moreover, there are even those who oppose Mr. Clinton's mild-mannered suggestion for *voluntary price restraints* on the basis that it eliminates cost shifting. All of this is particularly irksome when it is those self-same hospitals that have been piously assuring payers for over a decade that they *no longer cost shift*.

> **Politicians position themselves for re-election—and a great deal of misinformation is spread about every aspect of health reform.**

• All the lobbyists from the drug industry, the insurance industry, the medical "industry"—and even the AARP, the ethnic groups, and just about every other group in a country which increasingly is defining itself in terms of self-interested fragments rather than a cohesive commonwealth.

As if all this isn't enough to try the patience of a saint (and I make no claim to be one), there is the behavior of some nurses who tried to redirect deliberations at The National Nursing Summit on Health Reform. These fearless, forward-looking "nursing leaders" tried to introduce *entry into practice* as a relevant issue. As if this was not bad enough, they then did a lateral arabesque into the regulation of advanced practice. This meeting was called to solidify nursing's impact on health policy: an external issue. It was not called to deal with nursing's internal problems. It seems as if some people were born with their eyes glued to their navels.

Nonetheless and despite their incursions, the conferees resisted the temptation to fall into internal irrelevance and agreed on most of the major points of health reform. A new found unity was reached as all major nursing groups agreed to zero in on issues that are in the best interests of the public. It made me proud to be a nurse.

Now, to return to the point of this editorial—to wit, health reform—President Clinton sees most of the health purchasing alliances created by his plan becoming operational by 1996, although some states may not get them up and running until 1997—provided that the legislation passes this year. The employer health insurance mandate would take effect only as the alliances become operational. However, small business would not be affected until 1998 or beyond—and big business can opt out if it chooses, as long as the company provides the same standard benefits, plan choices or other provisions of the national plan.

The Republican party's response to the Clinton health reform proposal adopts managed competition but rejects employer mandates. With Clinton hanging tough on employer mandates, what potential compromise could be reached? Very likely the GOP may propose that employers provide a healthcare plan for employees but the employer would not be forced to pay for it—or at least not as much of it as Clinton proposes.

While state governors call for flexibility (and it looks like the Administration complied with their demand), and the Washington Business Group seeks as much national conformity as possible, various and sundry of our elected and honorable officials have introduced legislation that would augment, deter, or replace the Clinton proposal. What follows is a brief summary of what was introduced earlier this year:

Bill No.	Sponsor(s)	Date	Action
HR 101	R. Michel	1/5	• Malpractice reform, expands employer tax deductions, and insurance reform.
HR200	P. Stark & 66 co-sponsors	1/5	• Managed competition, global budgets, all payer provider payments, insurance reform.
S.325	N. Kassenbaum	2/4	• Sets uniform benefit package and annual limits on premium rate increases.
HR916	P. Stark	2/16	• Creates a board that would apply price controls to the Rx drug industry (*It couldn't happen to a more deserving group!*).
HR1200	J. McDermott & 87 co-sponsors	3/4	• Sets up a single payer system.
S.491	P. Wellstone & 5 co-sponsors	3/4	• Same as HR 1200.
S.572	D. Durenburger	3/11	• Allows the self-employed to deduct 100% of premiums.
S.728	M.McConnell	4/1	• Medical liability reforms, tax credits and vouchers for the uninsured and small insurance market.
HR2089	G. Brown	5/12	• Helps states set up Health Insurance Purchasing Cooperatives for small employers and the uninsured.
S.1057	J.Jeffords	5/27	• Managed competition with basic benefits package, financed by a 6% payroll tax.
HR2610	P.Stark	7/1	• Extends Medicare Coverage to all Americans.

In June of this year, the Robert Wood Johnson Foundation Survey on American Attitudes Toward Health Reform was released. At the very end of this lengthy document, the researchers conclude: "In virtually every respect, the debate over national healthcare reform is a debate about fairness. Americans believe that all citizens have a right to healthcare because that idea strikes them as eminently fair; likewise, the concept of explicitly rationing healthcare services, either throughout the population or just among the elderly, strikes them as inherently unfair.

> **Americans do not blame themselves for the problems of the healthcare system.**

"In a similar way, the public is currently averse to making major sacrifices in the name of health reform, because this too violates its sense of fairness. Burdens, they believe, should be assigned on the basis of blame, and Americans do not blame themselves for the problems of the healthcare system.

"They would, instead, fairly assign greater burdens to those they see as truly to blame: they would strictly regulate doctors, hospitals and insurance companies that they perceive to be wasteful and greedy, and impose higher taxes on those people, like cigarette smokers, who burden the system by creating their own serious health problems.

"Ultimately, then, the outcome of the healthcare debate will hinge on which side can seize the mantle of fairness and rally the American people around it. With so much at stake, all concerned will be competing furiously, trying to convince the American public that their position (and theirs alone) is truly fair."

In the end, then, the only question that really counts is: among all these proposals, "which is the fairest of them all—for me, for you, for the American public?"

November 1993

THE TSUNAMI EFFECT

"**Tsunami** (*n*), an unusually great, destructive wave sent inshore by an earthquake or a very strong wind." As a tsunami builds, it pulls water back from the shore; thus, it looks as if the ocean were drying up when actually it is building up. This is the tsunami effect: i.e., the drawing back, the perception that the market is drying up.

And this, I strongly suspect, is just where hospitals are today. Based on current occupancy data and extrapolations of HMO data, hospital planners are predicting a startling drop in the number of beds that will be needed in the future.

The problem with predictions

This situation reminds me of a pointed, if slightly scatological story my professor of epidemiology was fond of telling his *all-too-willing-to-distract him* students. According to Professor deGroot, New York City was a public health nightmare at the turn of the century: immigrants from Europe were arriving in large numbers daily, farmers *by the thousands* were coming into the city to find jobs in the factories, and the city's housing, transportation, sanitation and the like could not begin to keep pace.

Of all the desperate problems New York faced, a local columnist decided that the amount of horse dung on the city's streets best symbolized the sad state of affairs into which New York had fallen. "A lady may not even alight from her carriage without stepping into the odoriferous offal," the columnist noted.

Extrapolating data from a variety of sources—average increase in New York's population per year, average number of horses per 100 of population, average amount of dung produced per horse, average rate at which the sanitation department removed horse dung from the streets—he predicted that, by 1930, New York City would be two stories deep in horse dung.

There was nothing wrong with his data, it was his assumptions that were off base.... He assumed that the population would continue to grow at the same rate it had in the past 10 years.... He assumed that New Yorkers would continue to travel by horse.... He assumed that the sanitation department would not increase its efforts.... He assumed a lot of things—and none of them panned out. So, despite the accuracy of his data, his prediction couldn't have been farther from what actually happened.

The problem with data-based predictions is that they are always wrong...unless the *data* they are based on has been modified to reflect nascent technological, sociological, financial, environmental and philosophical changes. No matter how you cut it, data always represent the past—usually an artificially isolated segment of the past. And if there is an absolute, it is that all the circumstances which produced the past will never again be duplicated precisely.

> **Most of the oft-stated assurances that uninsured and under-insured Americans actually are receiving adequate care and treatment are based on political persuasion rather than public health information.**

And so let us return to the predictions of some of today's hospital planners. Considering the import given to their predictions, it is imperative to identify and examine the assumptions that underlie them. We already know about the data.

Looking at the assumptions

"**Assumption** (*n*), take to be true without proof." The "conventional wisdom" regarding much of the downsizing and some, at least, of the restructuring going on in hospitals today is based on the following assumptions:

Assumption #1—That almost all of the uninsured and the *underinsured* are receiving adequate healthcare—and certainly are being hospitalized, albeit grudgingly, today. That is why hospitals are losing so much money: the free care they have to give is bankrupting them. Therefore, the advent of universal access to health-care services will result in barely a *blip* in demand which will fall off at or below pre-reform levels.

Assumption #2—That, with or without reform, in the very near future, all inpatient care will be delivered under managed care contracts and that those contractual entities will be HMOs or HMO-like payors. That is why hospitals will lose money in the future: all care will be managed care and not only do hospitals lose on managed care contracts but there will be no place left to cost-shift.

Assumption #3—That current HMO bed-utilization data accurately predict the demand for acute inpatient beds in this coming universal access, managed care future. Of all forms of managed care, HMOs have the lowest inpatient utilization rates. Ergo, hospitals must downsize.

All of this, of course, is taken as true without proof: everybody just knows it.

It ain't necessarily so

Most of the oft-stated assurances that uninsured and underinsured Americans actually are receiving adequate care and treatment are based on political persuasion rather than public health information. Some because they think that *any other stance* will jeopardize the passage of universal access legislation (remember, conventional wisdom also dictates that universal access has to increase taxes, overburden employers and otherwise bankrupt the country). Others because they oppose passage of universal access legislation on the grounds that it is unnecessary, and the government always makes a bureaucratic nightmare out of things anyway. Still others because they are ideologically opposed to it: they believe that free enterprise is the most effective way—the American way—to make goods and services available to the public.

If they bother to cite a study to support their contention, it usually is the well-known RAND Study (a health insurance experiment) which found that coinsurance requirements motivate consumers to make wiser choices and reject frivolous services. However, a recent Office of Technology Assessment (OTA) study reports that co-payments—especially when the deductibles are high ($500 up) or the coverage is very limited (inpatient acute care only) or the patient's income is low—lead to "penny-wise, pound-foolish" health decisions. According to OTA, cost-sharing keeps people "out of the health-care system altogether."

And there are about 100 million of them.

Most of America's uninsured and underinsured population are not paupers; however, the vast majority of them have to think hard before exposing themselves to the kind of debt associated with today's health services. Take $1,200 for a lithium stress test for example. Or close to $1,000 for the average emergency room visit. Or $100 for a four-day supply of antibiotics. Or $670 to stitch a laceration.

Far from going bankrupt by providing free services, a recent PROPAC study indicates that hospitals are making more money than ever before!

The Clinton health reform bill would not change, or even threaten, the tax-exempt status of nonprofit hospitals, but *it would require nonprofit hospitals, for the first time, to perform yearly assessments of the healthcare needs of their communities and work with members of the community to address those needs.* Not a bad idea: one very close to the "social accountability budgets" proposed by the Catholic Health Association in 1989.

> **Rather than downsizing, we ought to be gearing up for the largest onslaught in history.**

If the underinsured are "being kept out" of the system, what do you think is happening to the uninsured? The good, decent hard-working folks who have something we can take away from them? The seriously-ill ones who have to measure their needs against their family's economic survival, or their children's education or their meager savings for retirement. The "worried-well" ones who may have something wrong, and who have to measure this "maybe" against the week's food budget.

And there are 38 million of them.

What's with the <u>blip</u>, Kemo-sabe?

Not only could there be more than a little *blip* in demand, there darn well could be a tsunami.... And it will be "unusually destructive" unless we start preparing for it now. Rather than downsizing, we ought to be gearing up for the largest onslaught in history. Rather than turning nursing units into mini-hospitals to attract the discriminating, we ought to be designing high-volume systems to maximize access by optimizing operations, equipment and personnel...systems that target high-risk patients and focus resources to minimize excess utilization...systems that will be humane even if they are not luxurious.

Certainly we will be moving as many services outpatient as possible. Yes, we will be developing subacute services and even whole subacute facilities. Of course we will be encouraging—if not downright forcing—families to take care of people in the home. BUT we are talking about adding more people to our health system than the entire populations of Canada, Australia, and England combined. And these "ADD-ONS" are likely to need some inpatient beds, even if their care is paid for through a HMO.

HMOs and their data

There are 540 HMOs in the country with a combined enrollment of 38 million people. Their ownership is about evenly split between for-profit and not-for-profit entities. By far, the majority of their subscribers are culled from the healthiest, lowest-risk Americans. Therefore, any data HMOs provide on resource utilization must be modified by this consideration.

However, once modified for a more general population, the data must be further modified by the fact that the U.S. population is aging. The outer edge of the baby-boom is now pushing 50 years of age. People over the age of 55 are about seven and a half times more likely to develop chronic, long-term or acute illnesses than those under that age. And they are likely to need a few more hospital beds than those younger than them. And no one seems to be taking these *facts* into account in their predictions of bed use.

Community hospitals and health networks will have to grow and expand: the huge tertiary care medical centers are the dinosaurs that must adapt or die. Government, business and individuals are beginning to change their value systems, and access to common health services for all is starting to eclipse the long-standing public fascination with highly complex, terribly expensive, incredibly esoteric heroic medicine. For one thing, our excesses in this regard taught the public that there are some things worse than death.

To put matters in a nutshell, universal access—under the Clinton plan—is likely to increase the growth of for-profit HMOs, hospitals and health networks. The impending merger of Columbia/HCA Healthcare Corporation is just one example of the frenzied pursuit of mergers and acquisitions currently underway. This is not a bear market, it is a bull market. So why all the gloom and doom?

Budget cuts and confusion

With all this talk about "reform," it's easy to forget that another round of cuts is included in next year's budget. While there will be some minor haggling about a few of its provisions, Congress is likely to pass the health portion of Mr. Clinton's budget with very few changes.

The relentless growth in Medicare and Medicaid not only consumes about one-third of the entire federal budget, but is blamed (and rightly so) for increasing the federal deficit. The Administration proposes Medicare cuts of about $118 billion next year by lowering hospitals' payment update, capital payments, and disproportionate share payments; eliminating hospitals' direct and indirect medical education payments; and cutting payments for outpatient services for starters.

The entire HHS budget is set at $673 billion, with the Administration's priority programs—child health and welfare, HIV/AIDS prevention and treatment, substance abuse, biomedical and behavioral research, family planning—getting funding increases and most other programs holding the line which, given inflation, is a funding reduction in real terms.

In the midst of all this, the American Medical Association (for those of you who have not heard this already) reneged on its promise to support universal access. It seems that the delegates were in a snarly mood last December when the House met—and the result undermines AMA's credibility with the Clinton administration. To further stir the pot, the American College of Surgeons, in a surprise move, not only embraced universal access but actually endorsed a single payor system. They are willing to cope with a Medicare-like system, but they don't want the hassle factor involved in complex, multi-tiered managed care systems—like Regional Health Alliances. This added support to the single payor schemes, especially Pete Stark's proposal to extend Medicare to all Americans. Meanwhile, American business, big and small, failed to endorse an employer mandate and demanded a market-based managed competition system. This gives more support to the bipartisan Cooper plan. Some expert observers of the political scene are ready to pronounce health alliances dead...which might be a bit premature.

Nonetheless, just about everyone in both parties thinks Congress will pass some kind of health reform legislation this year. And the President is determined to see to it that universal access is included, even if it has to be phased in gradually over several years. Appearances and experts and data notwithstanding, the tsunami is coming.

April 1994

Chapter 6

RESTRUCTURING: TRENDS AND ISSUES

HOSPITALS 1990: BACK TO THE FUTURE...OR ELSE!

It is not easy to care for the sick in a world in which the government makes one set of demands, and the public's expectations and values demand another. In a recent article in *Frontiers in Health Services Management*, Seay and Sigmond succinctly stated the problem "...current public policy toward hospitals implores them to act more and more like for-profit businesses, while chiding them for not acting enough like charitable institutions." Hospitals are being pressed to provide services to nearly 40 million Americans who have no insurance while state, county, and municipal authorities are "clamoring to find new revenue sources to restore federal cutbacks in domestic spending and to meet the demands of other pressing community needs."

In response, hospitals and health professionals have been striving for several years not to become more businesslike in their appearance, language and behavior. While federal reimbursement policies urge physicians to keep patients out of hospitals and compel hospitals to push patients back out fast if they *do* manage to get in, we have busily been working to convince the public that we're "big business": the health service industry.

Public discontent

The upshot of this unfortunate combination of factors is:

• A significant erosion in the public's confidence in hospitals and health professionals.

1. Robert Blendon, Chair of the Harvard School of Public Health, reported (1989) that "...89 percent of Americans see the U.S. healthcare system requiring fundamental change in its direction and structure."

2. Both Blendon and a recent Lou Harris poll report a steady decline in public confidence in medicine (from almost 80% to less than 40%) and hospital administrators (from 20% to about 15%).

3. A recent (September 1989) *Time* magazine article reported that 85 percent of Americans believe that physicians overcharge patients.

To an interesting and alarming degree, hospitals and physicians no longer are seen as benign and humanitarian dispensers of care. "Health Providers" are seen as merchants of life and death: those who can save life—but for a price, preferably paid up front. As healthcare increasingly has been depicted as a money-making industry, people are demanding greater value for money paid. Moreover, they expect their purchase of services to result in their satisfaction. Errors, mistakes and the general uncertainty regarding the results of medical intervention are less and less tolerated.

> **Hospitals and physicians no longer are seen as benign and humanitarian dispensers of care. "Health Providers" are seen as merchants of life and death.**

Threatened tax status

• The tax exempt status of the voluntary, not-for-profit hospitals is endangered.

1. More than a dozen states have re-examined, or have begun to re-examine, the basic tax-exempt status of voluntary hospitals as have many cities, counties, and other municipalities.

2. In Utah, hospitals must document yearly their benefit to their communities for the taxing authorities.

3. In Vermont, the city of Burlington—so far unsuccessfully—has tried to impose real property taxes on the Medical Center Hospital of Vermont. And in Pittsburgh local officials are systematically challenging the tax exemptions of the city's 17 hospitals.

Falling donations

• Donations to hospitals and to hospital foundations have declined significantly. After all, when was the last time you picked up your checkbook and wrote out a donation to one of the Fortune 500 companies? Many of our great medical centers were built on private philanthropy: gifts both large and small. People today are no less charitably inclined but charity for them is not—and never has been—defined in terms of profit margins and product lines.

To quote David M. Kinzer (AHA Leadership Project, Scottsdale, Arizona 1989) "...a major point of vulnerability... (is) that we have bought into the idea of becoming more 'businesslike' in our management, partly because we thought it would enhance our prestige. So far it has not.... While entrepreneurial behavior is being glorified in the hospital journals, our tax-exempt status is being threatened in Washington."

Transforming an image

The drive to transform the image of the hospital *back* to its charitable heritage goes far beyond fears about losing tax exemptions. From community reputation to litigation to fund raising efforts, hospitals need people to support them, to advocate for them, to work for—and within—them. The trend has been to "demarket" the poor; i.e., to hide from them in the hope that they'll go elsewhere for care; to transfer them (when they do find you) to public institutions ASAP; to dump them on the V.A. (a major reason why V.A. facilities will accept only patients with service-connected disabilities today).

This trend must be reversed rapidly—and the hospital's eleemosynary efforts must be made very high profile. Indigent care—social service centers, shelters for the homeless, soup kitchens—can and should be supported. Programs for the elderly—transportation, home meals, emergency medical response—should be widely publicized. Hospitals should not only support but seek to be identified with hospices, suicide prevention, cancer screening, child abuse prevention and treatment, children's health-care, rape crisis centers, poison control hotlines. Moreover, their sponsorship and participation in such programs should be carefully documented and recorded. And, I repeat, widely publicized. If it must be explained in business terms: supermarkets offer loss-leaders, and they're not even tax-exempt! There is nothing inherently paradoxical about hospitals providing compassionate reimbursed care to some, and compassionate free or subsidized care to others. To be both tax-exempt and successful, hospitals must be identified with their communities' needs, and within their communities as sources of responsive and competent care.

Bringing "old" values into the new world

Despite the inroads made by proponents of the industrialization of healthcare (as in healthcare industry) there are pockets of resistance among some old-timers—and a growing number of new-timers. Against all odds, they held their ground: health is a community service; hospitals are charitable institutions; doctors and nurses are compassionate caregivers. These indomitable, anti-industrialization guerilla fighters, brave last-ditch partisans of the "old" ways, never surrendered. While hospitals reorganized and diversified, these caregivers patted hands, talked to patients, consoled families and walked the extra mile with all who needed them. They can be found in housekeeping, dietary, x-ray, lab—and, yes, especially in nursing. They weren't fashionable for awhile and heavier workloads depleted their ranks, but in the end, they won. Caregivers must spend *time* with people (increasingly, the public is equating time spent with quality). And hospitals must *earn* their tax exempt status. And the public has to experience both. It's back to the future!

December 1989

STRATEGIC PLANNING: ASKING THE RIGHT QUESTIONS

"We belong to the ground. It is our power, and we must stay close to it. Or maybe we will get lost." Narritjin Maymuru Yirrkala, an Australian Aborigine, said these words. He spoke with a sense of purpose: of objective or intention. Of the ideal toward which one is always striving. Not merely a goal. A goal is limited: it is something concrete that can be achieved. It has a beginning and an end.

Purpose is bigger. It gives meaning and definition to decisions made and actions taken. Like giving excellent care to patients — Or meeting a community's health needs — Or serving the poor. Purpose is power, and without it organizations get lost. A sense of purpose lends *perspective* to decision making. And perspective is what strategic planning is all about. That is the first order of business.

The *second* is information gathering. In healthcare this includes: 1) identifying major areas of concern; 2) scanning environmental assessments from both the public and private sectors, 3) analyzing these assessments to discern major trends (nationally and locally), 4) synthesizing information to determine what changes are occurring within the health industry and 5) designing strategies for dealing with, modifying, and/or capitalizing on these changes.

Identifying concerns

While healthcare providers continue to struggle with cost containment measures, key issues are putting additional pressure on them:

1. *The economy*—Faced with recession, inflation and the threat of war, economic growth is expected to range from modest to stagnant. Public priorities are shifting from institution-based delivery of personal health services to improving the environment, handling addictions, preventing infection and controlling crime.

Thus, it is probably that government spending on healthcare will stabilize.

2. *Demographic changes*—The greying of America is the driving force behind changes in the style, type and content of health services delivery. As the number of persons over the age of 65 increases from 28.5 million in 1985 to 35 million in 2000 to 60 million in 2010, the demand for a wider *range* of health services is displacing the demand for heroic technological interventions. Of greater importance, however, are the baby boomers (fully 1/3 of the population). Their primary health concerns revolve around preventive care and routine illnesses, and their demands are focused on the development of convenient and personalized, if basic, care.

3. *Infectious disease*—A rapid growth in the incidence and prevalence of infectious disease is already beginning to strain the resources of the health industry. While the rise of AIDS (which is expected to crest in the mid-nineties) is the most dramatic, significant increases in tuberculosis, pneumonia etc., are of grave concern.

> **"Managing only for profit is like playing tennis with your eye on the scoreboard and not on the ball…"**

4. *Uninsureds and underinsureds*—Medical indigency is growing rapidly. In 1982, over 17 million Americans had no health insurance. That number grew to 38 million in 1988. This year it is expected to top 50 million. Disproportionate share hospitals are in imminent danger of sinking under the load. Competitive healthcare practices are making the situation worse. Public disillusion is reading an all-time high. Government is threatening the tax-exempt status of institutions which do not provide significant services to those who cannot pay. The possibility of national health insurance, universal coverage or even socialization is growing daily.

5. *The "bottom line" priority*—Excessive concern about and emphasis on improving the margin sacrifices long-term gain to

short-term profits. Blanchard and Peale in *The Power of Ethical Management* note that "Managing only for profit is like playing tennis with your eye on the scoreboard and not on the ball...[Yet] if you don't keep your eye on the ball, you won't get much on the scoreboard." No place is this more true than in healthcare. It is no accident that the new JCAHO nursing standards require quality data along with budget figures.

6. *Payor power*—Concern about quality in terms of *outcomes* will dominate payor initiatives in the next few years. Look for tighter precertification demands: quality care is *necessary* care. Look for tougher penalties for recidivism: quality care need not be repeated. Look for the development and *publication* of medical "practice options" (outcome standards). Prepare for hospital quality indices: quality care meets standards.

Scanning the environment

Six recent studies summarize trends that are shaping the future: *Seven Hospital Responses to Change*, the AHA 1989-90 Environmental Assessment; *Critical Condition: America's Healthcare in Jeopardy,* The National Commission for Quality Healthcare; *Nine Themes of Change and Uncertainty*, the AMA Council on Long Range Development and Planning; *The Trauma of Transformation in the 1990s: An Environmental Assessment of U.S. Healthcare*, published by Health One Corporation in Minneapolis; and *Looking Ahead at American Health Care*, Institute for the Future.

The meta-trends which emerge from a synthesis of their findings follow:

• the transformation of the hospital from facility to campus to concept. In the 90s, hospitals will become providers of total healthcare. Services will range from providing health insurance to case management to delivery of special diet meals-on-wheels.

• the transformation of the technological imperative from *using everything to ensure survival of a few to using what we have to improve the lives of the many.* Higher touch services will augment the move to less invasive technology.

- the transformation of physicians' leadership roles. Younger physicians are leaving their residencies to enter salaried positions, usually in physician-owned multi-specialty practices which contract for services with industry and health organizations alike. Changing expectations, payment schemes, and places of employment all alter the relationship of physicians to hospitals, health agencies and other professionals.

- the transformation of nurses' roles in service delivery. Critical pathways, skilled nursing assistants and technicians who report to staff nurses, professional nurse case managers and nursing HMOs—all evidence profound changes in nurses' roles. Legislative changes (advanced licensure, prescriptive privileges and the like) all underscore these changes.

- The strategies these meta-trends demand must fit the character and needs of each agency and community—which brings us back to perspective. After sharing information and analyses, take the time to determine what Blanchard calls the *Right Questions*, i.e., the questions which, if answered, will yield the best solutions possible. Then ask each member of the team "to sit quietly for 10 minutes and look for the answer to the Right Question(s) from within" (from Blanchard, K. and N.V. Peale, *The Power of Ethical Management*. New York: Wm. Morrow & Co., 1980).

I don't think we can stray far from our purpose if we take the time to think. Few of us really want to be remembered for the increment we added to the margin. Our purpose is larger. The integrity, intelligence and good will of most professionals will yield the right answers to the right questions.

To paraphrase Mr. Yirrkala: we are here to give patient care. This is our power, and we must stay close to it...Or maybe we will get lost.

January 1991

STRAIGHT FROM THE HORSE'S MOUTH...

The Chairman and Chief Executive Officer of the Prudential Insurance Company of America, Robert C. Winters, keynoted what the JCAHO has called a "landmark" conference, "Cornerstones of Healthcare in the 90s: Forging a Framework of Excellence." He began his speech with a story: "Recently," Winters said, "a Florida man had the misfortune to step on a splinter. He went to a local hospital to have it removed. He almost had to be hospitalized when he got the bill: $3,700. That's some set of tweezers!"

Thirty percent of care is unnecessary...?

Citing Winslow et al. in their 1988 study published in the *New England Journal of Medicine*, he quoted the following statistics: 65 percent of carotid endarterectomies were questionable; 56 percent of the indications for Medicare-reimbursed pacemaker implantations were either ambiguous or non-existent...and as much as 30 percent of the medical services delivered in the U.S. "may be unnecessary, ineffective, or inappropriate."

According to Winters, "physicians control the market and their decisions account for 75 percent of the costs...Some people get angry when you suggest that individuals other than physicians should have a voice in deciding what treatments are prescribed... Yet, how many of us are getting our money's worth? At the Prudential, we have invested $300 million in developing a national managed care network that will influence prices and treatments. CIGNA, AETNA, Travelers, Metropolitan, Humana and Kaiser are all doing much the same. Insurance companies are in a whole new business. We don't just write the checks anymore. We manage care. We approve providers, negotiate reimbursement, and screen hospitals. Our goal is to assess the quality and appropriateness of care."

The public: we've got to start somewhere...

Professionals' battles over the validity of measurement data won't be allowed to stop the march toward paying for patient outcomes rather than healthcare's process. Winters drove home the message from a recent *Pennsylvania Health Care Cost Containment Council* study, "A quarter of all stroke patients in one hospital died, while in a nearby hospital no stroke patients died. Now some people look at these numbers and call them meaningless... That data right now may not take all factors into account. But we've got to start somewhere. The Pennsylvania study found extraordinary differences among hospitals on price and success rates."

> **We must look at patient outcomes at different steps along the way. If the ultimate functional outcome is death, that's a little bit late.**

And start, they (and *we?*) are: in July of 1990, nine major payors met with the *Managed Health Care Association* and *InterStudy* to design a strategy for outcomes research. Moreover, the Feds aren't lagging far behind. The top priority for the newly founded (and underfunded) Federal Agency for Health Care Policy and Research is the development of medical practice guidelines. Many medical specialty groups have published practice parameters...and the development (and dissemination to the public!) of a hospital quality index is looming on the horizon.

JCAHO: performance data comes first...

Dr. Dennis O'Leary, President of the Joint Commission on Accreditation of Healthcare Organizations, summed up the conferee's growing consensus on comprehensively tracking providers' care effectiveness in these ways: "...Much of our discussion in this two-day conference has addressed different aspects of what I will call the "new evaluation tools" because that's what they really are: standards or guidelines, performance measures and large, new databases...The fact of the matter is that we must look at patient outcomes at different steps along the way. If the ultimate functional outcome is death, that's a little bit late. There are a variety of other intermediate measurement points about which we need information and for which we should have the ability to hold somebody accountable, if only to ask that previous performance be improved in the future.

"Not surprisingly, there seems to be a continuing comfort level with structural standards and structural measures," O'Leary said, "these include board certification or training that serves as a proxy for likely good performances. As performance data become increasingly available, we may eventually wake up to find out, for instance, that professional training and board certification don't make a large amount of difference. Quite clearly, the discomforts of the future are likely to revolve around being willing to acknowledge good performance without requiring that the performer have various tickets as proof of competence...No one disagreed that physicians and other practitioner groups must be intimately involved in development of performance measures and clinical standards...Interestingly, and I think, reassuringly, there was almost universal agreement that unnecessary and/or ineffective care should not be paid for..."

> **The name of the game is to prudently but expeditiously build a better mouse-trap...."**

Everybody's business: total quality management

Moreover, Dr. O'Leary continued, "Organizations will be using performance measures, they will be applying clinical standards and practice guidelines, and they will be engaging in continuous quality improvement efforts...the rational system of tomorrow will be a standards based system, but one that progressively emphasizes performance over structural requirements...This system will inherently say that one of the important jobs that must get done is to measure and monitor performance. Thus, there will clearly be a place for data—data that derives from good performance measures, data that professionals can believe...These databases will be crucial because isolated and fragmentary data, particularly in the case of small providers, of which there are many, will be of little use to provider or purchaser...

...Meanwhile, Dr. O'Leary concluded, "The Washington bureaucracy is taking a hardnosed posture. 'Yes,' they tell us, 'we understand that the methods we are using today are not very good, but we intend to use them until something better comes along.' That mentality is pervasive, and it has further raised the stakes. So the name of the game, in a very real sense, is to prudently but expeditiously build a better mousetrap...."

A word to the wise

The message for providers everywhere is clear. Gather your Q.A. data, track it over time, correlate it with financial indicators—budget, LOS data, recidivism. Do it now. Be ready to share it with payors. Read the "Report" published this month. Follow through. After all, we've brought it to you *straight from the horse's mouth!*

April 1991

WORK REDESIGN: OF SQUARE EGGS AND SORE HENS

Thomas Edison was fired from his jobs twice, both times for engaging in work redesign. Here's how he told the story himself: "The first time I was fired was when I was a telegraph operator. It was my fault, all right, but I got so interested in the dinged machine and its workings that I began to see how I could improve it. But I forgot all about the messages that were coming over the wire, and I left a lot of messages unsent and undelivered. Of course, they discharged me, and I didn't blame them" he added.

"Then," he laughed again, "I got a job in an office, and there were a fearful lot of rats; terribly old office, you know. I got up a thing that killed them like flies—the same with cockroaches. The floor used to be covered with dead roaches, and they fired me for that!"

The heart of redesign...

Improvement, not *necessity*, is at the heart of work redesign... although it is indeed true that necessity is the mother of invention. Problems of both costs and the shortage of nurses experienced in the late 1980s led to a variety of experiments in work redesign for nurses. In reading over—or looking over—some of the "redesigns," I got the feeling that their originators focused on cost to the exclusion of "improvement." Any legitimate work redesign will *improve* the product (in our case, patient care), the job or the conditions in which the job is performed.

Some of the other experiments in redesigning nurses' work seemed to me to be very different indeed, but not necessarily more efficient—and sometimes downright uneconomical. Thomas Edison never forgot his role as a businessman. When commenting on a newspaper article which described him as a scientist, Edison said, "That's wrong. I am not a scientist. I am an inventor..I measure everything I do by the size of a dollar. If it don't come up to that standard, then I know it's no good."

Not only must job redesign improve the "product," it also must be worth the cost.

Does it work...

Edison's school of scientific experimentation was essentially empirical. Once he was seeking a solvent for hard rubber. Many scientists, seeking it through theory or formula, met only with failure. Edison went to his impressive and remarkably complete storeroom of chemicals. He immersed a small fragment of hard rubber in a vial of each one of these many chemicals. Edison found the solvent.

Nursing is a discipline in search of a theory—or, at any rate, we have any number of theorists searching for one for us. Their propositions, especially when applied to the actual practice of nursing, must be tested empirically to see what "works" in more than theory. Never forgetting, of course, that the safety and satisfaction of patients comes first. For the most part, nursing and nurses are quite comfortable with Edison's school of experimentation. When we find something that "works" (improves patient care, saves time and resources and/or increases efficiency) we study it to "tease out" the theory behind it, i.e., those underlying truths which can be applied and adapted to fit other settings.

Learn to quit in time...

Job redesign is essentially an empirical venture. Don't be afraid to try something new...and don't hesitate to "chuck it out" if it fails. A triangular nest and square egg are no improvement over the old models. Moreover, square eggs make for sore hens—and sore hens think twice about laying any more eggs.

If you invest too much ego in a project you probably won't be able to let it go soon enough to prevent damage. Pride is the culprit, and patients are the victims.

But don't expect perfection

This is not, however, to infer that every new design comes out perfect the first time around. Edison, himself, had this to say about the invention of the phonograph: "I was working on the telephone, developing the carbon button transmitter. My hearing wasn't too good and I couldn't get the sounds as clearly as I wanted to, so I fixed a short needle on the diaphragm of the receiver. When I let my finger rest lightly on this needle the pricks would show me its amplitude and that's what I wanted to find out.

"One day when I was testing this way, it occurred to me that if I could indent a yielding substance with these vibrations, I could reverse the process and reproduce the sounds. I sat down and made a sketch of a machine that I thought would do the trick.

"Then I called in John Kruesi, my chief mechanic, and asked him what he would charge me for making it. He said he would make it for $30 and I told him to go ahead. Then he asked me what it was for, and I told him it was going to "talk." He thought I was joking and went away laughing.

"When he finished the machine and brought it back to me I put the tinfoil on, started her up, and recited "Mary had a little lamb." When I reversed and the words began to come back, Kruesi nearly fell over.

"That was the *only* one of my inventions that was perfect from the start."

In fact, when one of his assistants marveled at the bewildering total of his failures—50,000 experiments, for example, before he succeeded with a new storage battery—Edison exclaimed, "Failures! I have *no* failures. I learned fifty-thousand things that don't work: knowledge I put to use to find the one that *does* work." Patience. Persistence. Adjustment. Readjustments. Flexibility. Adaptation. *Willingness to reconsider.*

Quite possibly arrogance is the biggest obstacle to redesign. Oops, there goes another square egg!

January 1992

MULTI-SKILLED WORKERS: UNSAFE AT ANY PRICE

When I heard about *multi-skilled workers* (msws), each and every one of whom works for minimum wage and was trained in six weeks to do the jobs of eight or 10 paraprofessionals, I knew it was time to start explaining about *restructuring*. The multi-skilled workers I'm referring to here do not merely collect trays *and* mop floors. Golly gee, they do much more than that. You have to see it to believe it! These six-week wonders will practically *re-place* your phlebotomists, ECG technicians, pharmacy techs, IV techs, and x-ray and lab assistants. To round out their skills, they also can function as LPNs when they're not busy. Wow, they really are great! We should have thought of this before.

Hecky darn, these msws can help you turn each nursing unit into a mini-hospital. With most everybody but the RN earning minimum wage, administration can save 30-40 percent on personnel budgets alone. Moreover, patients never have to leave the units, well, almost never—not even the most ambitious consultants suggest you perform anything other than *minor* surgeries on the unit. Allegedly, patients will be so *happy* that the hospital's market share is bound to increase and with it, revenues will soar! To perform this little miracle, all you need to do is restructure your entire hospital around the concept of the multi-skilled worker...which will cost anywhere from $500,000 to $10 million in overhead and consultant's fees. And change the licensing laws. And the Joint Commission Standards. And fight the unions—or unionization attempts. And then there is always malpractice...But then, change is never easy—or cheap.

That's the price of progress. Right? Of course, some folks say progress means doing today instead of tomorrow what maybe we shouldn't be doing at all. However, with the U.S. House of Representatives trying to carve $50.4 billion out of the Medicare program over the next five years (that's $2 billion more than the President proposed!) and the Senate fixing to up the cut to $58.1

billion—not to mention the Health Reform legislation which hasn't even *hit* Congress yet—*something* has to be done. NOW. Fast.

A confidence game

Oscar Wilde once said, "Whenever a man does a thoroughly stupid thing, it is always from the noblest motives." I beg to differ. Ignoble motives can generate just as much stupidity. "Restructuring is often nothing more than a catchy sales slogan for junking yesterday's systems (and possibly its sanity) in the name of parsimony. The only thing progressive about it is the consultant's bottom-line.

Not, mind you, that I'm against "restructuring." Actually, I'm in favor of it. For one thing, it has historical grounding. All those who pushed for product line management should recognize it at once. So, for that matter, would Voltaire whose Dr. Pangloss repeated "Everyday in everyway, things are getting better and better" on the eve of the French Revolution.

> **Inevitably, costs are not *cut*, they are *shifted*.**

If someone believes a six-week training program can turn an uneducated worker into a multi-skilled wonder—or that a multi-skilled wonder would be willing to work for minimum wage if one could be so produced, the correct response is, "There's one born every minute."

Costs shifted not cut

The trouble with this sort of cost-cutting is that, inevitably, costs are not *cut*, they are *shifted*—whether we are talking about hospital "restructuring" or Medicare reductions. System-wide reform is needed, from the salaries paid to insurance executives, reportedly about $800,000/year—plus perks—to the President of Blue Cross-Blue Shield of New York, to the way we handle the uninsured.

In June 1993, the Prospective Payment Assessment Commission (Pro-PAC) released its report, *Medicare and the*

American Health Care System. ProPAC points out that, *despite* declines in hospital admissions and lengths of stay, hospital costs have risen once again to $832 billion in 1992—with a projected rise to $912 billion in 1993.

Hospital margins up

Though it's hard to believe, given all the yowling that has been going on, ProPAC further reports that hospital margins (excess of revenue over expenses expressed as a percentage of total revenues—business calls this a profit) are on the rise again.

In the first few years after PPS was implemented, hospital margins climbed to an unprecedented 6 percent. Subsequently, the Feds started clamping down on annual payment increases, and hospital margins did fall to 3.3 percent in 1988. However, that decline leveled off in 1990 and margins rose to 4.3 percent in 1991. In 1992, hospital operating margins increased again, and today they appear to be *higher than at any time before PPS was enacted.*

In all fairness, however, hospital's PPS operating margins (the difference between PPS payments and Medicare's portion of hospital inpatient operating costs) have declined sharply because operating costs for Medicare patients have increased faster than PPS payments. This fact, coupled with recurrent hints that health reform could be based on a one payor system, lies at the heart of many hospitals' urgent drive to cut operating costs.

Despite the Clinton administration's determined support of managed competition and thus, private insurers, providers fear the effects a *single payor* universal access system could have on their operating margins. And, beyond question, the "Single Payor" faction in Congress is growing stronger.

One payor "principles"

Rep. Jim McDermott (D-WA) collected 86 co-sponsors for his American Health Security Act (HR 1200) which ends private insurance and sets up a government-financed universal access system.

Although McDermott is realistic about the chances of his legislation being enacted into law, he thinks he has gathered enough clout to assure that the Administration's plan adheres to the following "principles":

- *Reduction* of administrative expenses
- *Comprehensive* benefit package
- *Single standard* of care
- *Freedom* to choose providers
- *Portability* of coverage
- *United* beneficiary pool (no link between employment and insurance)
- *Improved access* in rural and inner city areas
- *No barriers,* legal or structural, to a one-payor system

Reportedly, Clinton's plan calls for a four-year phase-in of universal coverage, a government-business partnership which includes the participation of private insurers, and the implementation of voluntary cost controls. However, the Administration has publicly acknowledged that its plan will allow the states to test single payor plans.

Status quo unacceptable

Beyond question, the Coalition of the Preservation of ERISA Preemption poses one of the most formidable barriers to state health reform. ERISA (The Employee Retirement Income Security Act of 1974) lets self-insured companies override state benefit mandates. Nonetheless, supporters of the *status quo* have a hard time defending their position. The U.S. spends more than twice as much per capita on healthcare as other industrialized nations. In 1991, the U.S. spent *per capita*:

- 50 percent more than Canada
- 67 percent more than Switzerland
- 73 percent more than Germany, and
- 74 percent more than France

Moreover, despite the fact that the U.S.A. does *not* offer universal coverage and had both fewer hospital days per person and the shortest lengths of stay of any industrialized nation, the U.S. also has the highest rates of growth in health spending.

ProPAC's report emphasized there is strong evidence that at least two cost-cutting measures *do* work. The first is rate regulation at least as it is practiced in Maryland. The second is managed care. We will see more of both.

Restructuring revisited

As healthcare reform comes center stage in the national arena this Fall, it does behoove hospitals to restructure:

Hospitals strong enough to resist fads and wise enough to plan change will be the winners.

• to determine how to meet universal demand

• to begin steadily reducing overhead as well as operating costs over three to four years

• to redeploy personnel as service sites and priorities shift

• to build networks of providers for expanding the services they can offer consumers

• to improve relationships with medical staff and among medical staffs and other non-physician providers so that efficient systems can develop.

Hospitals which find a way to keep the most competent people they have on staff; hospitals which cross-train workers to increase flexibility; hospitals which keep at least one eye on the services they provide (rather than both eyes on the bottom line); hospitals strong enough to resist fads and wise enough to plan change will be the winners.

There is time enough—and "margin" enough—to do it right. Any other approach to restructuring—especially one predicated on an undertrained and underpaid workforce—is unsafe at any price.

September 1993

BARBARIANS AT THE GATE

Quack, quack, quack. A row of ducks crosses the page of a pamphlet recently released by the Texas Medical Association. This unwise gesture is the latest step in a propaganda war intended to discredit nursing's advanced practitioners. Nurses' predictable response is anger at the injustice of the inferences and a new round of claims and counterclaims begin—all, of course, designed to inform/warn the American public. It is a sad and silly spectacle.

Advanced practice nurses have excellent safety records. Anyone who doubts this need only consult the actuarial records of malpractice insurance companies: the relatively low rates these nurses pay speak volumes. On the other hand, AMA has a point when it criticizes the educational preparation and credentialing of some advanced practice nurses—and nursing knows it. Katherine Chavigny, the nurse in AMA's Office of Nursing Affairs, presents AMA's position in a well-reasoned paper in this month's issue of NURSING MANAGEMENT. However, Chavigny's points may be swept aside in the fray over the "Quack, Quack" pamphlet.

The reason for all this sound and fury is that both professions are seeking to position themselves at the national level to "take over" primary care in America. The AMA claims that there will be more than enough primary care physicians—given sufficient public investment in their education—to meet the public's needs. Everyone agrees that there are not nearly enough of them today. The American Nurses Association claims that there could be enough advanced practice nurses to meet the public need for primary care in the very near future—given sufficient public investment in their education. ANA claims that advanced practice nurses, working collaboratively with physicians, can provide primary care less expensively and more effectively than physicians alone. AMA claims that nurses are willing to sacrifice the public's safety to their own ambitions as they seek to replace physicians.

Of barbarians and boards

Meanwhile, the "barbarians are at the gate" in tertiary care. The "barbarians" in this case are consultants and administrators—non-clinicians one and all—who are creating networks and systems for care delivery that effectively exclude clinicians from almost any input, no less influence, on major policy or resource allocation decisions. Take this scenario for instance: Under President Clinton's Health Reform proposal, Regional Health Alliances are to be formed. The Regional Health Alliance is a holding company: a company that owns/operates companies. The companies that it owns/operates are the health plans it must provide, at least a HMO, a PPO, and a FFS (a fee-for-service arrangement of some sort). Each of these plans is, in itself, a holding company consisting of the various provider groups, many of which are themselves holding companies. That is, "St. Elsewhere Hospital Corp., Inc." that reorganized and diversified in the 80s and may now consist of several hospitals, skilled nursing facilities, durable medical equipment companies, outpatient and even offsite pharmacies, home health agencies, diagnostic imaging and testing facilities, clinics, physician office buildings and the like. To further complicate matters, the holding company "St. Elsewhere Hospital Corp., Inc." may now be owned by still another holding company, "The Little Sisters of the Poor Multi-Hospital Corp., Inc."

Within this by-now-board-heavy-structure, St. Elsewhere is being restructured once again. Driven by not-unrealistic fears that one way or another managed care will cut margins (the nonprofit's word for profit) drastically, and dazzled by consultants' promises of saving as much as 40 percent of their personnel budgets, some administrators have not stopped at cutting to the bone. They are now dismembering their organizations and trying to fit them together in strange configurations. For example, nursing administrators are taken out of line positions and report to the CEO as staff. Most, if not all, of middle management has been eliminated. Unit managers, who may or may not be nurses and who may or may not even be managers (they may be lab techs or social workers or marketers), now control the nursing unit with, at best, a senior registered nurse to advise them. Staff nurses (some of whom have been replaced by "multi-skilled workers") report to the unit manager who, with no nursing background, is to staff, schedule, supervise and evaluate them.

Of imperial medicine and impotence

While nursing departments are being cannibalized, and nurses' ability to have impact on decisions and policies that affect patient care is being dissipated, physicians are struggling with their own crises. Unable any longer to deny the imminent demise of imperial medicine, many of them have entered Kübler-Ross' second stage of grieving—anger. And their anger blinds them to what is happening in the agencies and institutions within which they practice.

In an all-out effort to insulate themselves as much as possible from unwanted and hostile changes, they are making contractual arrangements with individual institutions which are parts of holding companies whose boards report to other holding companies (the HMO, PPO, or FFS) who report to yet another holding company (the Regional Health Alliance) Board. In such manner physicians' power and ability to affect decisions, including resource allocation, are diffused to the point of impotence. Thus, unless action is taken quickly, neither physicians nor nurses—in fact, no clinicians or only a token one or two—will be in policy-making positions.

How would we pay for it? Increase the Medicare tax. Wouldn't that cost too much? No.

While physicians and nurses face off over primary care, and hospitals seek to protect themselves from the incursions that managed care may have on their margins, the public debate over health reform continues unabated. Recent polls indicate that the President's plan, now introduced into Congress as the thirteen hundred plus page "American Health Security Act of 1993," is less popular now than when first introduced. This should surprise no one, given the millions spent by lobbyists and the self-interest groups to discredit and defeat it.

Of Congress, costs and one-payor plans

Meanwhile, back in the Congress, various one-payor schemes are growing in popularity—most notably Pete Stark's HR 2710 which, when combined with McDermott's HR 1200 with its 87 co-signers, bears a lot closer scrutiny than it's currently getting. What Stark is proposing is that Congress simply extend Medicare to cover all Americans. Medicare has been up and running for 25 years, and not only has it worked pretty well, we also know what needs to be done to improve it: rate controls, incentives for encouraging managed care, and for mandatory assignment for physicians for starters. Moreover, the rules and regulations are already written and approved: the "improvements" would require fine tuning the regs only. How would we pay for it? Increase the Medicare tax. Wouldn't that cost too much? No. The start-up costs would be negligible. Moreover, it could be up and running very quickly.

And past performance is very good indeed. Medicare and Medicaid now account for about 62 percent of the nation's health tab, but (and it's a very big but indeed) these two programs provide services for the two segments of the population—the poor and the elderly—who are at greatest risk of disease and disability: some seven and a half times greater risk than the remaining 38 percent of Americans. The privately insured (mostly working Americans and their dependents) and the uninsured (mostly working Americans and their dependents) are the healthiest segment—and thus the cheapest to insure segment—of the population. Last year, the non-Medicare/Medicaid portion of the population received care totalling about $340 billion. Medicare recipients' care cost about $215 billion. It is quite possible that the money saved by moving the privately insured, mostly healthy Americans, into Medicare would be enough in itself to cover care for the uninsured, mostly healthy Americans.

And political realities

Stark's proposal is seductively simple. Moreover, the Clinton Administration is not philosophically opposed to such a plan. So, while all the lobbyists and special interests are focusing on the Clinton plan, the Congress just might quietly pass legislation which extends Medicare coverage to all Americans.

Clinton's plan, on the other hand, would take far longer to implement, once passed, and the start-up costs could be gargantuan. in either case, no one today expects that any health reform legislation will pass before September of 1994. If the Clinton plan passes, undoubtedly with many modifications, all those 1300 plus pages would have to go to the Health Care Financing Administration (HCFA) to be translated into the regulations through which the law would be implemented. If HCFA managed to complete this chore in less than six months it would be a first class miracle, but let's say that HCFA does it. The proposed regulations would then have to be published in the Federal Register for 90 days to allow for input from the field. Let us now predicate another first class miracle and presume that no one objects to or obstructs the implementation of the regs.

The soonest the law could begin implementation would be 1995—and it has an extended phase-in period so that full implementation wouldn't/couldn't be accomplished before 2000. Too late by far to realize any savings, no less enough to keep health costs below the direful $1.5 trillion dollar mark. Too late by far to help reduce the Federal deficit. In short, too late by far to help in a reelection campaign. This alone might make the Stark proposal even more compelling to some.

All in all, 1993 has been a very interesting year, but 1994 promises to be a real donnybrook.

December 1993

LEARNING FROM THE FUTURE

The face on the cover of a recent issue of *Time* magazine did not belong to anyone. As the editor phrased it, "The woman on the cover of this special issue of *Time* doesn't exist—except metaphysically. Her beguiling, if mysterious, visage is the product of a computer process called morphing—as in metamorphosis, a striking alteration in structure or appearance." It was done to dramatize the results of interethnic marriage: her features reflect computer-blended characteristics of a person who is 15% Anglo-Saxon, 17.5% Middle Eastern, 17.5% African, 7.5% Asian, 35% Southern European, and 7.5% Hispanic. As a result, we can see the face of the future before it exists.

Whether "morphing" is performed by a computer, or accomplished simply by getting people together to brainstorm, its purpose is to create a vision of the future—one from which we can learn, one for which we can plan and prepare, or even one which we can change if we don't like what we see. It doesn't take a crystal ball so much as an open and *very* informed mind. For example, the computer expert, Kim Wan Lam, who produced this picture had to know a great deal about the current demographics of the country, the present and future trends in immigration, the physiologic traits of various races, the dominant genetic traits of each and how they would be likely to interact, and the willingness of people of various races, cultures and religions to intermarry.

Any vision of the future is composed of three elements: the past, especially in terms of those carefully collected bits of information called data; the present, particularly in terms of its trends; and the will of the people—not merely what *they want*, but what they are willing to work for and pay for (and what they are not!).

Don't count on the past

When predicting the future, most of us are *most* comfortable (and that isn't saying much) *most* of the time with a data-based analysis and projection. The problem is—and it is a serious one—that a purely data-based projection will *always be wrong*, not sometimes, always. Despite our comfort level with—in truth, downright fixation on—data, the fact is that data however carefully collected, catalogued and analyzed provide a very sanitized and limited slice of the *past*. And even if data from enough various sources could be synthesized to present an accurate picture of the past, any projection of those data into the future would be based on the assumption that all the conditions which produced the past would be duplicated precisely in the future: the only thing we know for sure cannot happen!

So, if our data-based projections are to be valid at all, they need not only be very broadly based, but also modified by an accurate analysis of current trends.

Don't be misled by the present

One of the most important things we can do to improve our ability to predict the future is to learn to distinguish a trend from a fad. A humorous, if unscientific, explanation of this process is that it is something like distinguishing between infatuation and love: it is difficult at first, but it's awfully important. A *fad* is a novelty: something new that catches our attention. We try it for a while and if it works, that is fine—and if it doesn't, we go on to something else.

> **With or without health reform, we are going to have managed care.**

One of the distinctive marks of a fad is that it is something we can adopt or abandon with impunity. It does not have deep roots.

A trend, on the other hand, has deep demographic, scientific, sociologic, financial and maybe even political roots. For example, *product-line management* in healthcare circles is a fad: if it works (and for the most part it doesn't), we keep it up. If it doesn't, we drop it and reorganize. It doesn't have deep roots and it doesn't make a whole lot of difference to anyone if it's changed. However, *outpatient surgery* is a trend which, even 10 years ago, could have been analyzed and recognized. Why? It has deep roots. Technology makes it possible. Financial savings make it desirable. Public acceptance makes it inevitable. It isn't just a way of organizing the hierarchy, it's a fundamentally different way of delivering services. If your organization did not prepare for the switch, it was a big loser. If it still won't retool for outpatient surgery, it won't be around long.

The same thing could be said about the move from private fee-for-service insurances to managed care. With or without health reform, we are going to have managed care. Why? Technology (in the form of computerized information systems) makes it possible. Every study ever done indicates that it helps contain cost, so financial savings make it desirable. And, considering the alternative which is fewer services—or no services for many—the public finds it acceptable. This combination makes it inevitable. So, if your organization is not gearing up to *capitalize* on managed care, if it isn't actively seeking managed care contracts, it will go the way of the dinosaurs. One healthcare leader even went so far as to describe yesterday's huge, technology/research intensive, inpatient focused university medical center as the medical equivalent of a *Jurassic Park*.

Don't discount the people

No matter what the data indicate, and no matter which way the trends point, what people want will have tremendous impact on the future, too. Make no mistake about it, what people want usually takes precedent in their decision-making over what they need, the only exception being genuine survival needs which supersede all else. Wants are not to be taken lightly, but they also must not be mistaken for something people think might be *nice* to have, but they really are not willing to work for it.

Ten years ago, for example, when DRGs first went into effect, a number of hospitals decided to focus their marketing efforts on those unlikely to be affected by them and those whose care was, by and large, lucrative, i.e., the normal maternity patient. They surveyed women to find out what they "wanted," and even offered options from among which they could select the most desirable. They did not, however, ask either the women or their *payors* if they would be willing to pay for these amenities. The upshot was that some hospitals spent millions remodeling their maternity units, installing jacuzzis and so on.

These plans, of course, were set in motion back when the *average* maternity patient had a 5-day length of stay and required little other than some teaching from the nurses. The trend among private payors toward cost controls was ignored. The demand for shorter lengths of stay was perceived to be limited to the Medicare patient. So, some hospitals made multi-million dollar bungles.

Others, while respecting the data provided by their past experience, and aware of consumer preferences, nonetheless took heed of current fiscal trends, and invested instead in birthing centers—and came out ahead.

Start with an environmental assessment

Developing an environmental assessment is essential to strategic planning. Any environmental scanning framework can be applied and adapted to each profession's or provider's unique marketplace or niche. I have found Health One's annual environmental assessment particularly helpful. (For a copy, write to: Health One Corporation, 2810-57th Avenue, North, Minneapolis, Minnesota, 55430-2496.)

Within this context, I would like to take a few moments to envision nursing's future. Our environment is unsettled to say the least. Everywhere in the country, nurses ask themselves and their colleagues, "Where are we going? What roles will emerge or expand? Will I have a job tomorrow—or two years from now? Is health reform only good for advance practice nurses? What is the future of America's hospitals?"

• *Where are we going?* With or without health reform, the U.S. healthcare system is moving rapidly toward managed care—if not managed competition. Institutional, agency and individual providers are forming health networks to position themselves to bid effectively for managed care contracts. Hospitals are restructuring and "right-sizing" (a euphemism for downsizing) to prepare themselves for continued moves to outpatient service delivery. Hospitals also are moving into long term care by capturing the emerging subacute market (a combination of skilled nursing, high-intensity home care, and rehabilitation) by converting some of their own acute beds to long term care beds, contracting with existing SNFs, expanding their rehab units and home health agencies, and developing linkages with their own DMEs and pharmacies as well as expanding the services they can offer by developing networks.

> **If your organization is not gearing up to *capitalize* on managed care, if it isn't actively seeking managed care contracts, it will go the way of the dinosaurs.**

• *What roles will emerge in the future?* Successfully gearing up for the future will require hospitals to have: 1) small (compared to their customer-base), flexible, highly productive workforces; 2) control of the outlier patient (the high-risk, high-utilization, multi-morbidity patient) and the outlier physician (those whose resource utilization significantly and routinely exceeds his colleague's); and 3) satisfied consumers (N.B., those who pay for as well as those who receive services are our consumers). Excellent, innovative nursing services help unlock the potential in all three key areas.

1. *Small, flexible, highly productive workforce.* For years nursing has talked about *differentiating* nursing practice. Patient-focused care offers the perfect opportunity. Nursing's associate degree nurses are ideally prepared to become the flexible, cross-trained, multi-skilled nurses who, on the nursing units, can provide—safely and with a minimum of on-the-job training—most services patients

need. This is particularly so if the nurse is paired with a cross-trained assistant who can provide the housekeeping, dietary, transport, clerical and other ancillary assistance the nurse needs.

Nursing's baccalaureate-prepared nurses are ideally suited to assume responsibility for developing the critical paths which improve consistency and quality, testing appropriate clinical and staffing standards, planning as well as supervising and evaluating the efficiency of the nursing services provided, and leading multi-disciplinary patient care teams in keeping with CQI objectives. With appropriate cross-training in management, they also are well-prepared to run clinical nursing units because their clinical knowledge enables them to assess staffing needs accurately, interact with physicians knowledgeably, and understand the problems of direct clinical caregivers clearly, *as well as* budget, assign, coordinate, and benchmark realistically.

2. *Control of the outlier patient.* Nursing's clinical nurse specialists are ideally prepared and suited to case manage the high-risk, multiple morbidity patient. Working in close collaboration with the many physicians ordinarily involved in the care of such patients, clinically competent case managers not only expedite care but improve its consistency and quality. And that, in our line of work, means the patients' care costs less *because* it is better.

3. *Satisfied consumers.* Patients and families are satisfied when the services they receive are safe. They are pleased when those services are provided by courteous, well-prepared and attentive staff. If patients also happen to meet with compassion and genuine caring, they may actually have been enriched by their experience and the hospital will have made a lifelong friend and supporter—and, this mortal coil being what it is, customer.

When care is given compassionately, competently *and* efficiently, it costs less. And people are much less likely to sue even if something inauspicious happens. This satisfies our other consumer: the payor.

Clinical competence enhanced by a service orientation is practically synonymous with nursing. Physicians know it: good relationships with the nursing staff is one of their prime satisfiers. Patients know it: patient satisfaction surveys have demonstrated the importance of nurses' attitudes and behavior time and again. The best administrators in the country know it: one of the characteristics of the *Magnet hospitals* is that the nurses were treated with respect.

- *What is the future of America's hospitals?* Hale and hearty. This is a difficult time of transition. However, with universal access to care looming on the horizon, all health providers can anticipate a significant increase in volume. Even though reimbursement per case will go down, the increase in volume will more than make up for it. Inpatient services *will continue to be in demand*, but growth will require an integrated network which includes:

  - offsite emergency services at several locations
  - offsite and ambulatory onsite surgical facilities
  - integrated subacute services
  - access to alternative and nontraditional therapies (acupuncture, biofeedback, chiropracty, massage, spiritual care)
  - high-tech diagnostic testing facilities
  - case management services
  - integrated benchmarking based on outcomes
  - health promotion, fitness, and health education facilities
  - telecommunication linkages to physicians' offices, patient homes, payors and regulatory bodies.

All this and more puts a lovely face on the future of nursing and healthcare. In fact, almost any *realistic* assessment of our future is remarkably rosy. President Clinton's *Task Force on Health Reform* even fretted that some hospitals would make *windfall* profits!

The only problem is "getting from here to there." Taking *what* we know about giving people care, modifying it by an accurate assessment of *current trends*, and wanting it bad enough to put aside turf issues so that we are able to work hard enough to "pay" for it isn't going to be easy. But, then, few things of value come easily.

January 1994

RESTRUCTURING: WHAT WORKS—AND WHAT DOES NOT!

We trained hard—but it seemed that every time we were beginning to form into teams, we would be reorganized. I was to learn later in life that we tend to meet any new situation by reorganizing. And what a wonderful method it can be for creating the illusion of progress while producing confusion, inefficiency and demoralization.

Gaius Petronius Arbiter
First Century A.D.
As cited in *Satyricon*

In the face of fierce competition for managed care contracts, many hospitals are reorganizing—engaging in cost-driven downsizing, down-staffing, labor rollbacks, and elimination of services. And they don't even know if it will work. In the Spring of 1993, E.C. Murphy, Ltd., published the findings of a two-year study designed to assess the effects of restructuring methods on HCFA Medicare-reported mortality data for hospitals.

The study, involving 281 general acute care hospitals, found a strong relationship between mortality in Medicare patients and cost-driven downsizing. Specifically, "hospitals that made across-the-board staffing cuts of 7.5% or more...or who were at an average staffing level of 3.35 FTEs per adjusted occupied bed or below...were more likely to experience an increase in mortality and morbidity."

The study also found that inefficient systems in the typical hospital "force" employees to waste almost one-third of their time. Moreover, the average hospital spends *only 31 cents of its labor dollar on direct patient care*. However, this figure does not take into account the waste factor; therefore, the typical hospital actually may spend less than 22 cents of its labor dollar on direct patient care.

Murphy's findings support those of other researchers. According to a study published in the *New England Journal of Medicine*, hospitals with more registered nurses on staff and higher ratios of nurses to patients had 6.3 fewer deaths per 1,000 patients than hospitals with fewer nurses and lower nurse-patient ratios. More than a dozen studies show that hospitals with higher ratios of registered nurses to patients have lower mortality rates, shorter lengths of stay, fewer complications, and thus lower costs.

What is the mission?

In the Nov. 18, 1993 *New England Journal of Medicine*, Dr. Arnold Rellman warned that "All present signs indicate that most plans will be owned by insurance companies or other healthcare businesses [like pharmaceutical companies?]...eager for a share of what promises to be a huge and profitable market."

And the competition is savage!

If the mission is to capture 'a profitable market,' then restructuring focuses on eliminating unprofitable services, buying professional practices, and eliminating competitors.

I had always thought (hoped) that a hospital's mission was a great deal more than "capturing a market." I thought that a hospital's mission was to help the ill regain their health.

If this is the mission, then restructuring will focus on assessing community health needs, designing services to meet them, and optimizing professional roles. In any case, successful restructuring efforts must start with a clarification of the organization's mission—who *are* you, what do you *want* to become, and *how quickly can you safely get there.*

Restructuring, reengineering and job redesign

Before any changes are undertaken, you need to answer two questions: *In light of our mission, what are we doing right?* and, *In light of our mission, what are we doing wrong?* The answers should be organized according to the following:

Restructuring, which involves the architecture of an organization. Generally, restructuring advocates prefer managerially lean, decentralized, self-governing organizations that empower first-line caregivers to make decisions.

Reengineering, which has to do with revamping the *processes* by and through which things are accomplished. "User friendliness," efficiency and economy are the watchwords.

Job redesign, which deals with who should be doing what, where, how much and for how long. Flexibility, cross-training, and productivity are essential.

If Murphy is right, and hospital workers spend 31% of their time trying to overcome inefficient systems, then downsizing will overburden workers unless the hospital reengineers its processes to eliminate wasted time. Similarly, downsizing and cross-training are effective only if the personnel whose jobs have been redesigned are able to do the work.

The work to be done

If the work to be done is patient care, then the data show that the best person to do the job is a well-prepared nurse working in an empowered and respectful atmosphere. As early as 1986, researchers at George Washington University found that the quality of nursing care is the most important factor affecting the survival rate of patients admitted to intensive care units. Using the APACHE II scoring tool to measure patient status and predict deaths in 13 hospitals, the researcher found dramatic differences in mortality ratios:

- In hospital 1 (hospitals were numbered according to mortality ratio), the predicted number of deaths was 69; the actual number of deaths was 41.

- In hospital number 13, the predicted number of deaths was 33; the actual number of deaths was 52.

- In the best hospital, the nurses had protocols to follow that permitted them, within expertly defined limits, to make minute-to-minute changes in adjusting respirators, administering blood pressure control drugs and so forth. They also had the authority to cancel elective surgery when needs exceeded nursing resources. Relationships with physicians were excellent, and communication was both frequent and mutual.

In the worst hospitals, i.e., those with the highest mortality ratios, nurses were constantly pushed to accept more patients than they believed they could care for safely, they had little or no autonomy, and communication was poor.

Nurses and physicians working together *can* effectively reengineer patient care delivery, as New England Deaconess Medical Center demonstrated with the development of *nursing critical paths*. By amalgamating nursing and medical care plans, identifying the nursing interventions required at critical junctures, specifying what outcomes were expected from the interventions, and putting it all on a time line, they increased both the quality and consistency of patient care, and thus reduced costs.

This is reengineering where it counts, i.e, where most costs are incurred, at the bedside.

Outside the walls into the networks

Originally, professional nurse case management was conceived as a way to improve the quality of care by creating an organizational structure that would allow the best prepared nurses to remain in sustained contact with the most complicated patients. It soon became evident that to capitalize on the concept, the care—and thus the nurses—had to move out into the community; thus, Ethridge et al. developed a Nursing Network. The results were published in 1989: Length of stay went down, and inpatient acuity went down as community-based nurse case managers facilitated early intervention, which either prevented rehospitalization or brought the patient back into the hospital at a lower level of acuity.

In short order, the nursing department spun off a "nursing HMO" that contracted with a medical HMO to deliver nursing services to its 10,000 clients over the age of 65. The result: Within three months, the nursing HMO saved the medical HMO about

$700,000, principally by reducing inpatient days. Now, THAT is restructuring!

UAPs and the cost of care

Over 25 years ago, Luther Christman published careful studies of the use of nursing assistants in hospitals. To put the matter in a nutshell, he found them to be the *most expensive workers in the hospital.* One can almost hear Luther proposing such "Ironclad Laws of Management" as:

1. The lower the educational level, the lower the pay.
2. The lower the pay, the lower the morale.
3. The lower the morale, the higher the use of benefit time.
4. The lower the pay, the lower the morale, the higher the turnover rate.
5. The lower the educational level, the lower the pay, the lower the morale, the greater the need for supervisory time.
6. The less the education, the lower the pay, the lower the morale, the higher the risk of accident and error.
7. The higher the risk of accident and error, the greater the liability.

The U.S. Army has been very successful in using unlicensed assistive personnel. It calls them Medics and trains them for a period equivalent to that of a licensed practical nurse. However, civilian UAPs provide services ordinarily delivered by personnel from dietary, housekeeping, lab, pharmacy, physical therapy, transportation, radiology, I.V. therapy, ECG and nursing. And *they* are *not* trained well.

According to McLaughlin and Thomas (*Nursing Economics,* April 1994), who surveyed California hospitals on their use of unlicensed assistive personnel, 88% of hospitals provided less than 40 hours (one week) of classroom instruction, and 99% of hospitals provided less than 120 hours of on-the-job training for newly hired UAPs. So the average UAP receives less than one month of combined classroom and on-the-job training.

Nonetheless, the hospitals spent $3,800 to train just one UAP. Moreover, of all the hospitals surveyed, only one reported using multiple measures of cost-effectiveness such as cost per length of stay, turnover, and quality assurance monitoring.

The heart of the matter

So, what works and what does not work? We have a few answers:

- We *know* that restructuring hospitals to facilitate professional nurse case management on the continuum works, if by working you mean increases patient satisfaction, improves patient outcomes, and saves money.
- We *know* that reengineering (implementing critical paths) works—if by working you mean increasing the consistency and continuity of care and decreasing costs.
- We *know* that physician/nurse collaboration works—if the APACHE II studies mean anything at all.
- We *know* that cross-training works—provided the cross-training falls within the scope of the person's educational background and experience.
- We *know* that nurses can move services out into the community, and that patients, physicians and payers love it.

We *know* what doesn't work, too. Poor communication, low morale, too few nurses for too many patients, too many assistive personnel for nurses to supervise, *and* down-substitution do not work—if by *not working* you mean patient morbidity and mortality rise, turnover increases, unionization grows and liability increases.

Hospital restructuring, reengineering and redesign WORK, and work well, only when nurses are enabled to *practice*, and to practice well.

October 1994

UNSAFE PATIENT CARE: THE ROAD TO ABILENE

Some years ago a young man, who later became very influential in the development of management theory and practice, went to Texas to visit his bride's parents. His in-laws lived on a farm just this side of nowhere: it was 100 miles to anywhere from where they were. They arrived during one of the worst heat waves that part of Texas had experienced in 10 years, so folks weren't doing much. On Sunday afternoon he found himself sitting on the porch playing dominos with his wife whilst they sipped lemonade and basked in the breeze of an electric fan. His mother-in-law was sitting on the porch swing. His father-in-law strode onto the porch, took a swig of lemonade to clear his throat, and said, "How would you like to drive into Abilene for dinner tonight?"

In part to break the uncomfortable silence that greeted what she considered an insane suggestion, his wife said, "Perhaps the young people *would* enjoy going out to dinner." The young man who, after all, did not want to offend his new in-laws, said, "Sure. That sounds like a great idea." His bride, anxious to please him, and unwilling to be the only one to say "no," hastened to add, "I love to go out to dinner!"

So, they clambered into the old Ford and started off for Abilene. The temperature was a scorching 110 degrees Fahrenheit.

The car wasn't air conditioned, so the windows were wide open, letting all the dust from the road fly in through them and settle on the hot, sweaty bodies inside. It took about two hours to reach Abilene, and when they arrived, all the restaurants were closed because of the heat wave: most everybody was home on their porches drinking lemonade and sitting in front of their electric fans. A half hour later, they finally found a greasy spoon that was open. After a thoroughly unsatisfying meal that none felt like eating because they were too hot and gritty, they climbed back in the car and drove another two hours across scorching highways to get home.

Plopping herself back down on the porch swing, the mother-in-law snarled, "That was just about the stupidest thing we've ever done!" Her husband snapped back, "The only reason I suggested it was that I was afraid the kids were bored just sitting around—and *you* agreed with me!" "Don't blame it on us," the bride said defensively, "We only went so we wouldn't hurt your feelings."

Years later, when he was trying to figure out how once-successful organizations made stupid decisions that endangered or even ruined them, the by-now-not-so-young man remembered the trip to Abilene. And he used it to describe the phenomena that he observed. He called it "The Abilene Paradox": i.e., no one wanted to go to Abilene, everyone thought it was a stupid idea and yet everyone supported the suggestion...and the whole family went to Abilene. The utterly predictable failure of the trip engendered anger as each blamed the others for the misery they suffered. No one told the truth, and each felt justified in his/her lie.

...is paved by team players

This pretty well sums up the situation in health care today. Everyone had better be a "team player," and team players support one another and they support management: criticism is negative, and negative people don't last long in today's job market.

A staff nurse in a California children's hospital told her supervisor that she thought the staffing levels were unsafe, and the next day she was "laid off," allegedly a victim of restructuring. Whether or not this story is true (and I have faith in the veracity of the nurse who told it to me), anecdotal evidence gathered from every part of the country indicates that criticism leads to elimination. If this is the case, a great many hospitals could be well on the way to Abilene!

While commitment to a change is necessary, falling in love with it usually spells disaster because if you do, you'll want to implement it everywhere—even when it is inappropriate. When you fall in love with a certain approach, you are unable to see its failings—and you will "kill the messenger" if anyone tells you about them. Moreover, you are incapable of seeing the merits of alternative approaches. What is even worse is that the state of being in love is, by definition, irrational. Some have even called it temporary insanity. Demanding "blind commitment" from all team players is neither rational nor enlightened: it is both despotic and counterproductive. And effective managers have known this since theory Y challenged theory X.

...who have survivor's syndrome

Considering the enlightened state of 20th-century management, how could such behavior occur at all, no less be "widespread"? In his book, *Healing the Wounds*, David Noer proposes another theory that could explain some of what is going on in hospitals today. He uses the term "survivor syndrome" to describe the psychic condition of those who remain employed in an organization that has been downsized. The more rapid and brutal the cuts, the more serious the illness. "Survivor sickness" dulls the moral sensibilities, which leads to behaviors that, in all probability, diminish the chances of an organization's survival.

Harvey Eichman calls survivor's syndrome "marasmus" (Gr. "wasting away") and lists among its symptoms negative self-image, low self-esteem and low energy, all of which contribute to low morale. Just about every productivity study ever done links low morale with low productivity. If this situation is not addressed, the organization soon becomes as dysfunctional as its members. In health service delivery, this situation can be very serious indeed—and employees and organizations are not anywhere near as endangered as patients and families.

...which threatens patient safety

Quality assurance experts are concerned because there is a dramatic drop in the number of incident reports nurses are filling. Although it is *possible* that no untoward events are occurring, it is unlikely that this is the case, especially in view of the rapid changes that are occurring and the inevitable morale problems that accompany downsizing even when it is undertaken with great sensitivity. What is far more likely is that nurses are not filing incident reports because they are afraid they'll be fired if they do file them. Why are the QA people concerned? Because they do not know what is going on, and thus they will not be able to track and correct problems. This, in turn, is giving risk managers nightmares.

It also makes it very difficult to assess the effect that various restructuring efforts are having on patient care. Identifying problems, tracking incidents, and making mid-course adjustments is especially important in light of the role changes being piloted in many organizations today. In his book, A Whack on the Side of the Head, Roger von Oech notes that "Your error rate in any activity is a function of your familiarity with that activity. If you are doing things that are routine for you, then you'll probably make few errors. But if you are doing things that have no precedence in your experience or are trying different approaches, then you will be making your share of mistakes."

When you are changing routines, trying new delivery systems, introducing new skills, you should *expect* errors, and thus the number of incident reports, to rise. This is as inevitable as it is unintended. Errors should be anticipated, tracked and corrected. According to von Oech, they "serve a useful purpose: they tell us when to change direction...we learn by trial and error, not by trial and rightness." If people will not report errors because they are afraid of the consequences, we are well on our way to Abilene. If employees are too burned out from "survivor's sickness" to care enough to report them, we've not only reached Abilene, we may die there.

What can be done?

There are some signs that hospital management has "fallen in love" with an idea, or perhaps that "survivor's syndrome" is spreading like a virus through the healthcare industry. If you are "in love," you'd better fall out of love very quickly or you will soon be:

- buried in liability (after years of remaining flat, malpractice claims are on the rise again)

- battling a union (SEICU alone has managed to win union elections in Las Vegas, Syracuse, Buffalo and Tacoma in the last few months)
- explaining to your Board of Directors or Trustees just why you lost a managed care contract because of your recidivism rates (recidivism is on the rise nationwide).

If you can honestly say that you are not "in love" with a program, concept, project or idea, then look for the signs of "survivor syndrome." Successful organizations take into account the emotional aspects of change similar to Kübler-Ross's Stages of Death and Dying: denial, anger, bargaining, depression, exhaustion, acceptance and finally ownership.

Different managerial tactics are appropriate at different stages:
- counter denial with reiteration of the changes and the reasons for them
- confront anger and explore its source with employees
- listen to the bargains but do not compromise the changes
- anticipate the increased use of benefit time that comes with depression
- plan on decreased productivity during the exhaustion phase
- look for the first signs of acceptance, which usually are characterized by nostalgia for the good old days
- be prepared to adopt employees' suggestions during the change to cement the "buy-in."

In any case, and for whatever reasons, no hospital can afford to lose the active participation and honest reporting of committed health professionals. At the moment, managed care is still on the increase and driving down costs seems to be the only thing that matters. But soon—very, very soon—there will be a shake-out, and the unsafe providers will be the first ones to go belly-up. Driving costs down without tracking and measuring its effects on patient care is a one-way road to Abilene. No one wants to go there, and we will avoid it only if someone can and will tell us the truth. Unsafe care isn't a bargain at any price.

January 1995

COMRADE HEALTHCARE WORKER...?

Not long ago, I walked into a hospital, went to the information desk and was greeted by someone named "MARY healthcare worker." Following "MARY healthcare worker's" instructions, I found the inpatient unit which housed my friend Jane. As I entered the unit, "JOAN healthcare worker" was performing an ECG on Jane. A short time later "JOAN healthcare worker" cleaned the room, took Jane's blood pressure, delivered her food tray and gave her some medications. During the visit, Jane mentioned that "SUSIE healthcare worker" seemed to be running things, but she wasn't sure. "You can't tell *who* anybody is around here, and you can't figure out who you can ask about what, or who knows what," she said.

On the way out, "JOHN healthcare worker" helped me find the way when I took a wrong turn. I noticed that "JERRY healthcare worker" was clipping the bushes. Later that afternoon, I had an appointment with my own physician for a routine checkup so I asked him about this "healthcare worker" craze. He said, "I hate it. I can't figure out who's who. It's confusing as #*@!"

"Hmmm," I thought. "The patients don't like it and doctors hate it. This is really strange." With curiosity thoroughly piqued, I called a few nursing colleagues who worked at this hospital. One said, "Management's just trying to hide the fact that there are so few nurses left in the place anymore." She was not a happy person so one might be inclined to discount her remark, but even so I had to admit that if I'd seen a nurse, I didn't know it.

Another colleague said, "It's a quality thing. See, if no one has a title then everyone is equal, and we'll all work together better. It's sort of like a classless society." "I see," I said, "We have '*comrade healthcare workers*'. How interesting." Pure egalitarianism did not work under communism, so we're trying it again under a capitalist system.

What's in a name?

Absolute equality did not work for communism simply because everyone is not absolutely equal—in brains, education, ambition, skill, dedication and the like. People *are equal* in the eyes of God. People *are equal* under the law. People deserve an *equal opportunity* to succeed. But that's about it when it comes to equality.

The philosophical basis of a capitalistic system is that those who are more talented, those who work harder, those who produce better results *are rewarded* with money and status. It is called a career open to merit.

We did not beat the communists, their system collapsed from within because it was so inefficient: one of the major reasons why is that people were not rewarded for their work. People *need* to identify with their work, to take pride in it and to be recognized for it.

Respecting persons doesn't mean you wipe out their differences. Respect for names, titles and personal and professional identities is not foreign but rather integral to team building. You really can have a quality organization characterized by effective team efforts *and* still allow individual team members to have—and to be known by—their professional identities...with all the baggage that entails—licensure, statutory limits and authority, ethics and the like.

The melting pot theory of team development—NOT!

Since when do you have to eliminate professional titles, ignore professional competencies and blur professional roles to create an effective team? One might call this the melting pot theory of team development. This approach allegedly is based on principles culled from TQM (total quality management) and CQI (continuous quality improvement). Some see it as essential to radical restructuring and job redesign. And, as is the case with most radical ideas, it is intensely idealistic and naive.

If you want to run an effective anything, you have to respect human nature: what it will stand and what it won't. Many years ago, when Marxism was making inroads in Scotland, a Scottish physician by the name of George Cheyne defeated his communist opponent with the following words: "Hoot, hoot, man! Human nature is a rogue and a scoundrel, or why should it perpetually stand in need of laws and of religion? A man won't willingly give away the money he's earned or the title that's his by right. Your high ideals sound fine to the ear but they willna' work."

The loss of professional credentials and titles demoralizes those who hold them—particularly those who worked the hardest and sacrificed the most to earn them. The following situation illustrates the point: *At the age of forty, Maryjane found herself divorced with four children to support. With less than $20 per week child support from her ex-husband (and even that was less than reliable), she entered the job market. After a frustrating series of minimum wage jobs, she decided that her only real hope for a decent future for herself and her children was to go back to school. She worked hard and she studied hard, and there were times when she was so broke she didn't have money for toilet paper. It took years, but she made it. At her graduation party, she held up her diploma and she said, "This is mine. I earned it and no one can take it away from me!"*

Imagine her dismay when someone does take it away from her, when she becomes a generic "healthcare worker"—all in the name of egalitarianism, no less.

Professional identity personified...

Professional identity isn't a matter of feeling superior to someone else. Being a nurse—or a physical therapist, or a pharmacist, or a social worker—is part of who one is. Being recognized as a nurse in one's place of employment helps one get the job done far more efficiently.

Moreover, the accomplishments of the members of "my" profession help me to define my role more clearly, provide models of behavior worthy of emulation and, whether or not I pause to notice it, give me a sense of affiliation—of belonging to, and being responsible for and to, something greater than myself.

This is not to deny or belittle the contributions that members of other professions have made—or that those employees who are not members of any professions have made. It certainly is not a bar to working closely with people of other professions, vocations or job titles.

However, this does infer that members of a profession answer to others outside the internal "chain of command" in any institution or agency:

- to the public in the form of the individual persons to whom they give care;
- to the statutory body that licenses them to practice;
- to the profession, upon whose pronouncements many of their legal and statutory obligations are based.

Professional responsibilities and team activities...

This does not mean that professionals cannot be effective team members. It does mean that their employers are not completely free to define what is and is not in the professionals' role—nor can employers, acting alone, divvy-up the legal, statutory or ethical duties of professionals among team members who do not belong to that profession.

It does not mean that professionals cannot delegate certain responsibilities to others. It does mean that they—along with their employers—are responsible for the correct performance of these responsibilities. *Respondeat superior* does not mean that the employer is the only one liable, it simply means that the professional's employer *is also liable*.

Having, in fact cherishing, a professional identity does not mean that professionals cannot be loyal to both employers and to other team members. It does mean that their first loyalty is to the person(s) upon whom they lay hands—and that "loyalty" is defined by the public in the form of statutes, rules and regulations as well as case law; and by the profession of which they are members in terms of codes of ethics and standards of practice.

Defining an effective team...

If the communist experiment taught us anything at all, it taught us that human beings yearn to be seen and recognized as individuals...that morale (and thus productivity) are *enhanced* when people are recognized and rewarded for their contributions...that human nature can be ignored only at your own peril. Therefore, the use of a generic title is more likely to harm quality than enhance quality.

If, on the other hand, my cynical colleague is correct, and the elimination of titles is undertaken to hide the paucity of professional expertise on staff, then it's nothing but a swindle: it cheats staff and it cheats the public.

There is a famous story about an old man, his wife and the local rabbi. The old man and his wife were inveterate gardeners and could be found working the soil morning, noon and night. Each day as the rabbi walked to his office, he would admire the Goldstein's garden. "Mr. and Mrs. Goldstein," he'd say, "You have a beautiful garden. You and God are partners." Every night as the rabbi walked home from his office, he would see the Goldsteins still working hard in their garden. "Mr. and Mrs. Goldstein," he'd say, "You have a beautiful garden. You and God are partners."

This went on for years, every morning and every night. Finally, Mr. Goldstein could stand no more. One fine evening he answered the rabbi, "It's a good thing God has us for partners. You should have seen how this placed looked when He had it alone!"

Teams, like partnerships of all kinds, do best when each member is clear about her/his role and scope of authority, secure in the knowledge of who she/he is, and aware of the contributions each person brings to the achievement of the team's goals.

Excellent teams do not require the creation of the "comrade healthcare worker." They require people who respect one another, which is quite another matter altogether.

April 1995

Chapter 7

NURSING AND SOCIETY

Nurses: Bimbos on the Boob Tube?

The year was 1983, and it was impossible to find an October issue of *Playboy* magazine. Why? Because it featured a 10-page display on "Women in Nursing." Naturally, hardly anyone read the few words which surrounded the pictures. The article actually wasn't bad: it spoke of nurses' new responsibilities and higher education, of nurses' struggles and ambitions and varied roles.

I first became aware of this outrage when, following my verbal rendition of the American Academy of Nursing's Public Relations Committee report, Anne Zimmerman asked, "Mrs. Curtin, what are *you* going to do about *Playboy*?" Another distinguished nurse said, "I've never been so shocked! No nurses I know look like the women portrayed in those photographs!" Feeling was running high, and nurses bought *Playboy* magazines by the carload, and wrote letters to its editors by the bushel. The gist of those letters was that nurses are hard working and devoted to their jobs. We wear flat shoes and starched pinafores over our flat chests. Certainly nurses are devoid of any of those attributes so brazenly portrayed in *Playboy*. "Visit your local hospital," we challenged them, "and you will not find one nurse who bears any resemblance whatsoever to those nurses in *Playboy*."

> **There *is* a different, demoralizing quality about how nurses are portrayed...**

Nurses don't waste their spare time cavorting about boat docks and night clubs. They attend educational programs on their days off and spend their evenings reading nursing journals. Why, I know hundreds of nurses who have turned down dinner dates because they'd rather study blood gases at home than sit around a candlelit restaurant holding hands with some attractive man. When a woman goes into nursing, she takes a vow of chastity, and promises to devote all her waking hours to carry out the nursing process. Nurses are a breed apart—selflessly dedicated and loyal to their employing agencies. They would as soon think of failing to complete a nursing care plan as of posing in the buff for *Playboy*. Sooner, in fact, *Playboy's* outrageous exposé only played into the hands of those sexploiters who use nurses to profit the medical-industrial complex.

So the argumentation went and so it still goes.

The nurse as sex object

Ever since a couple of sociological studies showed that the entertainment media portrays nurses as sex objects, nursing's "image problem" has focused almost exclusively on the sexploitation of the profession. Nurses' indignation is almost knee-jerk predictable: "We are *not* sex objects" we proclaim. To a certain extent, this concern, while overstated, is valid. However, it seems to me that just about everyone in the entertainment media is a sex object...And this state of affairs isn't anything new either. I can remember rushing back to the dormitory during my student years to watch *Ben Casey, MD*—and it wasn't because he was a doctor. As I matured, *Marcus Welby* started looking pretty good (even though his "nurse," Carmen, *was* a bit of a twit), and nowadays even George Burns gives my heart a little flutter. In all honesty, can any of you claim that the officers on *Miami Vice* have no sex appeal? And what about those lawyers on *L.A. Law*? If they're all "sex objects" too, why should nurses complain? Nonetheless, there *is* a different, demoralizing quality about how nurses are portrayed...

The nurse as utter incompetent

It wasn't until I had an afternoon appointment with an orthopedic surgeon that I was able to identify the difference. This is what happened.

My physician, having studied Medical Economics 101, routinely schedules about 55 patients every 15 minutes. Not surprisingly, patients usually have a long wait during which they watch the waiting room television set thoughtfully purchased to distract them from their discomforts. Ordinarily, patients negotiate among themselves to determine which program they want to watch. Our group of patients voted—and I lost 54 to 1, so we watched *General Hospital.*

The scene opened in a patient's room. The patient was a handsome young man about the age of my oldest son (22). He was lying in bed with a sheet stretched over his manly chest and tucked up under his dimpled chin. Although I did my nursely best to do a thorough physical assessment on this young man, I could find nothing wrong with him. The nurse was a—shall we say mature—woman, at least my age. (My fellow patients informed me that her name is Jessie and she's the head nurse.) This nurse was the picture of the "modern" RN: she wore a tailored dress, full-length lab coat with a stethoscope draped gracefully around her neck, and she wore three inch heels.

It was difficult for me to determine *what* Jessie was doing in the patient's room. She did fluff his pillow on several occasions. Otherwise, she minced about the room (in all fairness, one cannot stride purposefully forth in three inch heels, about all one *can* do is mince) and carried on what, in my day, would have been called a "suggestive" conversation.

In the midst of all this mincing, fluffing and suggesting, the patient went into a cardiac arrest. What do you suppose Jessie did about this patient emergency? Did she do what any self-respecting sex object ought to do...i.e., snatch the opportunity for a little mouth-to-mouth? No. She didn't even do what your average American visitor would do..i.e., put on the bell and yell for help. Jessie abandoned the patient and minced quickly out of the room, screaming for some character by the name of Dr. Hardy. At this dramatic moment, the episode ended. A brief inquiry elicited the information that Dr. Hardy was the Chief of Staff. Then I knew the kid was doomed—by the time someone found "The Chief," he'd be very dead indeed.

The nurse as competent, compassionate contributor

Owing to the fact that I'd another hour to wait before I would be seen, I had plenty of time to think about nurses, nursing, *General Hospital* and how Jessie portrayed us. Did it bother me that Jessie clearly had a "thing" for a man young enough to be her son? Was that the problem? Or was the problem that a senior "member" of my profession was portrayed as panicking in the face of a patient emergency, abandoning the patient and screaming for someone else to help? As the mother of three erstwhile boy scouts, let me assure you, the youngest of them would have behaved better. They would have started CPR...but a registered nurse runs away?

> I do resent it when nurses are portrayed as bimbos on the boob tube: that hurts— and it undermines the credibility of the profession.

The real problem isn't that nurses are portrayed as sex objects, but rather that nurses are portrayed as *nothing but* sex objects.

Ben Casey was a sex object, but he also was the best doctor who ever lived. He was doing heart transplants in 1960—on Tuesdays. On Wednesdays he did brain surgery, on Thursdays he delivered babies in the ghetto! He was interested, concerned, competent, compassionate, committed—and making a difference in the world. The cops on *Miami Vice* may be sex objects but they risk their lives to help people, and to make our world a safer, better place to live. The lawyers on *L.A. Law* fight the whole system to defend the rights of the oppressed and correct injustices—and, by the way, they have families and lovers and sex lives which they routinely mishandle.

I have no objection to being a sex object (go ahead America, eat your heart out). I don't mind if people want to think nurses are beautiful and desirable and even sexy. But I do resent it when nurses are portrayed as bimbos on the boob tube: that hurts—and it undermines the credibility of the profession.

Reinforce the positive images

If we nurses wish to affect how nurses are portrayed in the entertainment media, we should write...but write only when nurses are portrayed as competent, compassionate human beings who make a real difference in the world. Receiving letters—getting attention from the public—is a reward for the media. It's smart to reward behaviors we want to see repeated. It's easy to write when you're angry, but it's more effective to write when you're pleased.

On February 28, 1990, organized nursing launched a major campaign to enhance the image of the nurse. Very soon we should start seeing more and more positive ads, stories, and portrayals of nurses. The campaign needs, nursing needs, the media needs reinforcement to continue. Nurses of America, write on!

May 1990

MARIA'S CHOICE

How do you take the measure of a man—or a woman? Sister Maria is 75 years old. She is about 4'10" tall and weighs 72 pounds. She has a moderately severe scoliosis of the spine, osteoarthritis and rheumatoid arthritis. She has survived multiple surgeries and a major stroke. Her right shoulder is dislocated. Her jaw has been shattered in a fall—so badly that it cannot be set. She's been mugged seven times at last count.

She suffers more pain than almost anyone I've ever met.

And she's the only one I know who visits a young man convicted of hacking his foster parents to death. Sister Maria started working with street people years ago. Long before it became popular, she struggled to find housing for the homeless. She visits shut-ins, and reads the works of the most contemporary—and often most controversial—theologians. She's usually good for a handout, but she's nobody's fool. If you need food, she's likely to give you a check made out to a local grocery store. Only the uninitiated are deceived by Sister Maria's soft voice and gentle ways: she is a strong woman. A woman of principle. A woman of prayer. A determined woman indeed!

This is her life, and this is how she chooses to live it.

Pain, limited motion, digestive problems, and more pain interfered with her choices, with her living. Finding ways to control the pain and build her strength meant that Maria could go on with her life. It now means that she can work six to eight hours a day, six days a week.

Sister Maria is a woman who "spends" her health. She spends it on things that are more valuable to her than health itself. Sister Maria, and other patients like her, give us a different perspective on health. Health for them is a personal resource, a capacity which enables them to express their values and sense of purpose. By almost any measure, Sister Maria's life is "healthier" than that of many people who are physically fit—and purposeless. She is a woman who chooses to live by her values.

In doing so, she presents her caregivers with difficulties. The stronger she gets, the more she works. The more she works, the greater her stress. The greater her stress, the greater her pain. She wants to be alert, so she rarely takes pain medications or sleeping pills. The less she sleeps, the weaker she gets. The harder she works, the greater her stress, the tireder she gets, the greater her pain. To keep her going is to keep her working. Often in dangerous areas, or climbing on buses or walking the streets. But "to keep her up and doing" is to enable her to use her life. That not only gives her personal satisfaction but also the opportunity to meet needs she sees as greater than her own.

> **Caring is to healing what curing is to survival.**

Lives like Sister Maria's are rare, but are patients like Sister Maria so uncommon? People do value things which enhance the meaning of their lives more than they value health. Few people make health their life goal. Health is a means to an end, not an end in itself. Health is not the goal; living is the goal...not life itself, but rather the *living of a life*. Life's "trade-offs" are common—and commonly missed. People often choose to get less sleep than they need, skip a meal, or work long hours under stress in order to do something which is important to them.

Any fair examination of today's healthcare delivery system will conclude that it focuses on survival. Simplistically put, curing is the goal: an understandable and good but an insufficient end.

Illness and death surround health professionals with pain. Nurses and physicians in particular are "confronted daily with the vulnerability of the human condition, a vulnerability which professional training sensitizes them to detect. Professionals are also confronted daily with the full spectrum of human strength and resilience which they are not as systematically trained to see. Without the ability and skill of seeing the latter, the former may become overwhelming and so painful as to cause people to withdraw and distance, to protect themselves in ways that make them smaller and less alive than they should be." (Remen, Naomi. *The Human Patient*. Anchor Press. 1980, p.183-184.)

And patients get efficient, technical service. Sometimes it is even polite. Patient and family are left alone with the illness to follow directions—or not. Usually they go on living, sometimes all the way through life to death. Perhaps because of our perspective, we stay focused on their survival. And we burn out.

The most significant questions health professionals can ask themselves are, "Do I serve *surviving* or *living?*" "Is health really physical fitness or the patient's capacity to respond to her inner direction and her sense of larger purpose?" If so, in daily interactions with patients, the professionals' guiding principle should be the affirmation of the person's life and the support of her growth. The denial of death and the preservation of bodily function are subordinate to the person. Therefore, professionals must *consciously* acknowledge the context of their work—to see themselves as working in relationship with people rather than as acting on people. Working in relationship *with* people *is caring*. Its function is healing. Indeed, caring is to healing what curing is to survival.

We've already discovered that surviving without healing is appalling. What we have yet to learn is that there is no real curing without caring. Compassionate concern makes people feel that they are understood, not as they seem to be, not as others judge them, but as they are. Every person is important—special, unique—and each one's living is more important than our knowledge, turf and technology. That's the message of caring.

If living is the goal, then our greatest health problem today is that people don't think they are special. We acknowledge their specialness when we share their goals. Thus, even when we may not cure them, our caring still can help heal them. Sister Maria walks the streets again. And she's already been mugged seven times and she'll wear herself out and she'll do as she chooses. That is health. And that, after all, is why we're here.

December 1990

...Of Alligators, Ants and Fireflies

Professionals in general, and nurses in particular, tend to shroud their opinions discreetly in careful qualifications. Such precision and reticence undoubtedly are commendable in journal articles and scientific seminars. However, they make editorials boring. They tend to leave the reader with the bland (and non-threatening) impression that on every issue there is much to be said on both sides and in every content area, more research is needed. I tend to favor non-technical language like "fat rats" over "obese *ratti*," and the danger of "assertion" over the security of "waffling." One of the attitudes to be fostered in nurses, too long conditioned by authoritarian teaching, is that they don't have to agree with everything they read in the literature. In fact, half the fun of living is in challenging (rather than swallowing) what you read.

...which brings me to my real concern—you.

You are the person who delivers service in an overbusy world, who manages in a changing world, who feels endangered in an uncertain world.

You are alive. You are in a precarious state. Life itself is a physiologic tightrope with death on either side. To stay alive you must maintain yourself within a narrow range of temperature, electrolytes, blood sugar concentration, metabolic rate and so forth. Let's focus on only one of these factors—temperature.

Nature has decreed that your temperature should be 98.6 degrees F. Some variance is tolerable, but with a little too much or a little too little you die. You have certain physiologic mechanisms for maintaining your temperature at the optimal level, despite variations in the temperature of your environment: if the temperature is too low, you shiver, if it's too high, you sweat. Now consider the alligators of the swamp, how they survive: they shiver not; nor do they sweat. Even Solomon in all his glory was not alive like one of these. Why do not alligators die of fever or hypothermia? A group of alligatorologists received a grant (no doubt, a federal grant) to find out. They traveled to Africa to discover that, when an alligator is too warm, it slides into cool water; when it gets too cold, it climbs onto a hot rock. That is, the alligator maintains its optimal temperature by adjusting the environment to itself, rather than by adjusting itself to the environment. Human beings do both.

You are employed. You are in a precarious position. For the most part, a professional's career is a footrace between obsolescence and retirement. To stay employed, you must maintain yourself within a narrow range of knowledge, skill, political ability, humility, self-esteem and so forth. Let's focus on only one of these factors—self-esteem. It is not uncommon today to open a newspaper and see an announcement of more healthcare cuts, and of hospitals reducing services or even closing their doors. Such announcements engender apprehension, fear and insecurity among healthcare workers. Unfortunately, fear and insecurity breed poor decisions at best and cruelty at worst. Those who retain their feelings of security do so because these feelings are genuine and rooted in the bedrock of self-confidence. Security is not found in things or organizations—it is a feeling about oneself. It is derived from one's experience of oneself: one's ability to be of service, to earn, to produce, to think, to enjoy. Unlike alligators who mindlessly borrow their temperatures from their environment, human beings can adjust their temperatures by keeping their inner poise. They do not allow themselves to be blown away by uncertainty and fear.

They develop self-confidence by living each day to the fullest. Learn to be concerned about *today*. Set a goal—and meet it. Don't allow rumors or fear about the future to take over. Set aside a "worrying time" each week. And keep your worries for that time. List them. If they aren't real, dump them. If they are real but outside your control, set them aside: they're someone else's problem. If they're real and within your control, write down what you plan to do about them. Do it.

Do something for yourself and your staff to build security: educate against obsolescence and use "downtime" to envision new futures. Foster personal habits which elicit confidence: *Presence* ("walking around" versus sitting around or distancing oneself from personnel); *Poise* (command presence has something to be said for it in times of stress); *Purposefulness* (make the mission visible, follow through, "be there").

Learn to be unconcerned about things you can do without. When professionals express concern about their security, they don't really think they are going to starve, or go naked or die of exposure. For the most part they are concerned about their possessions, position and status. Take inventory of the way you live, the money you spend, the possessions you have acquired. How important are they? Important enough to devote your life to them? Important enough to be a prisoner of fear for them? To be unkind or cruel to others in order to keep them?

Accept the rules of living. You are alive, and life itself is a hazard. No guarantees come with life or with a career or with a job. When you feel insecure, you are refusing to accept the risks of living...and your fear will do nothing to eliminate your risks. Plan your future, build your abilities and live in confidence. Take care of your mental and emotional self.

Stay loose. Get a body massage. Learn to watch ants. Thoreau learned a lot from them. Plant wildflowers. Cry during movies. Invite someone dangerous to tea. Send yourself flowers. Take lots of naps. Believe in magic. Laugh a lot. Draw on the walls. Go skinny-dipping. Listen to old people. Read books. Take walks. Hug trees. Swing as high as you can on a swing set. Write a love letter. Take moon baths. Listen to the music you like. Sing out loud. Dance. Drive away fear. Play games. Celebrate a gorgeous moment. Give money away. Do it now. Build a snow fort. Chase fireflies. Say something nice to someone. Set aside a time to dream. Do it for love. Surprise yourself.

Take good care of you. People need you. You need you.

February 1991

HEALING THE SPIRIT

Perhaps the pendulum finally has swung in the opposite direction. The greedy eighties seem to be giving way to a more aesthetic nineties. People today hunger for personal healing and spiritual growth. The signs—aftermath of the spiritual devastation of the eighties—are all around us. Consumer magazines publish articles about the "downwardly mobile": those yuppies who found that material success did not yield personal happiness. Wary of formal religions, the young and old alike nonetheless seek the comfort of spiritual companions.

A vicious circle

The pervasive disease of the nineties is essentially spiritual. Self-abuse—ranging from co-dependency through the addictive disorders all the way to suicide—is common. As a matter of fact, the more we learn about disease (from lung cancer to ASHD), the more we realize that many diseases are life-style related, i.e., a result of our own choices. Self-destructive choices.

Other-abuse—ranging from child molestation through elder abuse all the way to murder—is on the rise. As a matter of fact, the more we learn about other-abuse, the more we realize that it stems from self-abuse which in turn stems from shame, i.e., a result of early victimization: abusive choices made by others.

Generalizations lead to minimization

A bewildering array of literature, professional and popular alike, suggests all kinds of reasons and even more solutions to these problems. Often the literature, while giving a nodding bow to probable relationships among and between co-dependency, addictive behaviors, depression and guilt, nonetheless ends up treating each as a discrete problem...and often seems to expand the scope of each to extreme ends. For example, if one reads the "co-dependency literature," one is left with the impression that anyone who is even polite to someone else is co-dependent. If one reads the "guilt literature," one is left with the notion that guilt is always destructive (isn't there anytime when one ought to feel guilty about one's slimy behavior?). The addiction experts leave one thinking that anyone who enjoys an ice cream cone is an addict. Health professional and patient alike are afflicted. Everyone is "sick"...So, our generalizations lead to minimization and, in the end, we ignore the pain—and the abuse continues. The most neglected, least understood and least addressed dimension of healthcare is the healing of the spirit—the healing of that intangible union of physiological, psychological and subjective elements that comprise what Martin Buber called the human *dasein*. We yearn for an "I-those" relationship with someone which, in turn, would enable us to develop an "I-those" relationship with ourselves and with our world. To accept, respect and cherish the special, vulnerable, fragile, wonderful human person. You. Me. Us. Them. We.

What happened to that vulnerable child who opened his or her eyes on the world and took it all in? Violated? Wounded? Protected? Aggressive?

In need of acceptance, integration and healing. And, in the healing, we are made whole again. Then, we, in turn can support others in their own healing—for ultimately, self-abuse can only be "cured" by self-healing.

From encounter to integration

In an attempt to organize and rationalize the information bombarding us on all sides, I found (and I don't even know the source) a model that helps explicate the relationships among the various steps—and barriers—to healing the human spirit.

A traumatic encounter occurs—perhaps it is physical or sexual abuse—usually in life. This experience generates shame: I am not worthy of consideration. The pain of unworthiness is masked by co-dependent behaviors in which we sacrifice our own needs to the needs of others. And the first barrier to healing is set in place.

If one actually acknowledges the wants and needs generated by the trauma, the feelings this generates may result in addictive behaviors which hide or deny these feelings. Almost anything is preferable to feeling the pain.

Once experienced, the pain often generates anger which the person (especially if the person is a woman) may judge to be "wrong." Thus, it is suppressed and turned inward on the self. The result is depression: the most common disease in the United States today!

If the person can be helped to identify this anger, express it clearly, and focus it on the appropriate source, she is well on the way to accepting her needs, wants and feelings: to accepting herself. The single most formidable barrier to self-acceptance is guilt. Guilt because you have been shamed, because you have stood up for yourself, because you have acknowledged your anger. Thus suggesting that you are worth something. And, especially, guilt because you have focused that anger on someone else—often a significant other. If the guilt can be overcome, the experience can be integrated. And with the integration, the human spirit is healed.

About nurses

The nursing literature suggests that many nurses are co-dependent. So much so that one is led to believe that co-dependency is a requirement for entry into the profession. In my mind that's going too far, but I do believe that nurses—just as all other people—can be hurt. That nurses need healing, too. And that it's not only okay, it would be wonderful if we could support one another through the process. Perhaps understanding what is going on can help us help ourselves, help one another and eventually help our patients/clients to heal. The healing has to start somewhere. Why not with nurses?

December 1991

LESSONS FROM THE STEEL AXE

For over one hundred years, sociologists have studied the collapse of the Yir Yoront society. The Yir Yoront were an Australian aboriginal tribe who supported themselves primarily through hunting and fishing. The stone axe was their primary, all-purpose tool.

It also had great cultural significance. Only men could own an axe. In fact, only men could even *make* an axe. Should a woman need to use an axe for any reason (preparing food, chopping wood, etc.), she could borrow one according to prescribed rules of kinship. The kinship rules reinforced the privilege associated with masculinity, and the power of the patriarchal family.

Toward the end of the nineteenth century, European missionaries arrived bringing with them steel artifacts including the steel axe. The Yir Yoront women, in particular, welcomed them and worked for and with them. In return for their labor, and in well-intentioned attempts to ease their domestic workload, the missionaries gave the women steel axes.

Women who have no option but to flee find that isn't much of an alternative either.

Because those steel axes were superior to the stone ones, the Yir Yoront men wanted them, too. However, they would not work for the missionaries since it was not in keeping with their dignity or their customs. Therefore, they had to borrow the steel axes from women—a significant role reversal. The ownership of a stone axe lost its symbolic importance, and the construction of stone axes lost its association with masculinity.

Family and social relationships were disrupted. Power was redistributed. Some of the women even flaunted their steel axes. Men felt emasculated: some began to blame women for their turmoil. Eventually, a victim of backlash, the tribe disintegrated.

Contemporary backlash is growing, and the fear that fuels it has frightening implications. Faludi's recent chronicle of the crumbling status of American women (*Backlash*, Crown Publishers, Inc., New York, 1991) is only one example, but it is a powerful one.

The tale of the Yir Yoront is a metaphor for late 20th century American society. There are many lessons to be learned from it. To the extent that we understand the cultural, technological and sociological forces at work, men and women can avoid the fate of the Yir Yoront.

The product of fear

A backlash is a product of fear. That fear is a normal human response to social change. The social change is occasioned by technological advance. Such advance in itself changes, sometimes even reverses social, domestic and work relationships. Backlash does not arise from deliberate conspiracy. It is far too pervasive and subtle for that. It is driven by economic transformation.

Centuries ago, Fernan de Rojas wrote, "It is safer to be despised than to be feared." Why? Shakespeare said it all in *Antony and Cleopatra*, "In time we hate that which we often fear." And, in ancient times, Cicero wrote "Hatred is inveterate anger." And Petrarch wrote, "Anger is brief madness and, unchecked, becomes protracted madness, bringing shame and even death."

These observations are all too true. Since the early '70s, rapes have more than doubled and sex-related murders increased 160 percent between 1976 and 1984. Between 1983 and 1987, domestic violence shelters recorded a 100 percent increase (*Backlash*, XIX and XX).

Faludi puts it succinctly "...in 30 states, it is still generally legal for men to rape their wives, and only 10 states have laws mandating arrest for domestic violence—even though battering was the leading cause of injury to women in the late '80s. Women who have no option but to flee find that isn't much of an alternative either...one-third of the one million women who seek emergency shelter each year find none [an interesting though perhaps unrelated fact makes this situation even more poignant: at least one-third of women who are murdered, are murdered by their husbands or boyfriends usually just after they filed for divorce or left home]...almost half of all homeless women (the fastest growing segment of the homeless) were refugees of domestic violence."

Violence against women is only the tip—albeit an ugly and intimidating tip—of the backlash iceberg. The really widespread effects of backlash are far more subtle.

Women in the workplace

To return to the Yir Yoront metaphor, the steel axe changed their lives. Technology is changing our lives. And no one is going to go back to the stone axe again.

For example, beyond question, the computer is one of our most powerful tools. Not only *can* women use one as well as men, but often women *in the workplace* learned to use computers *before* men did so. In fact, as we look at contemporary tools of work, there are few if any "tools" that women cannot use at least as well as men. The "old tools" required episodic use of physical strength. Modern tools require persistent agility. It's like the difference between splitting rock and knitting. Many modern tools are actually more suited to the physical and emotional characteristics so often attributed to women.

The public economy far more than the women's liberationists have drawn women from the home into the marketplace. The notion that "the little woman" works for fun or strictly for luxuries is as demeaning as it is untrue.

Perhaps the worst part of all this is the implication that women *choose* to work, while men *must* work outside the home.

> **The worst part of all this is the implication that women *choose* to work, while men *must* work outside the home. Therefore, it is all right, in fact it is necessary, to discriminate against women in the workplace.**

Therefore, it is all right, in fact it is necessary, to discriminate against women in the workplace. Faludi notes that CEOs of the Fortune 1000 companies (80% of them) admit discrimination in the workplace affects their female employees. Even so, less than one percent of these CEOs regard remedying sex discrimination as a goal their personnel departments should pursue.

Thus, the average female college graduate still earns less than the average male high school graduate. And the average female high school graduate earns less than the average male high school dropout. Moreover, at least 80 percent of full-time working women earn less than $20,000 a year—twice the male rate.

Nonetheless, women are working while there are men who are out of work, so the threat is there. And, because the tools have changed, the fear is there, too. The fear is that women will supplant men—rob them of their status and their roles.

The technological revolution has changed workplaces and job requirements. No amount of anger, no amount of discrimination, will change this. Ever since the industrial revolution, men have tied their identities to their jobs, and measured their self-worth by their ability to earn money outside the home. Earning a living for the family symbolizes masculinity. It is the stone axe.

Technical competence is the contemporary steel axe.

Until men understand this, they will blame women or women's liberation for social and economic problems. Until women understand this, they will not be able to overcome the backlash. Until both sexes understand the metaphor, we won't be able to develop the new symbols and new paradigms necessary for stability.

March 1992

Good Intentions Pave the Road...

Those of you who are among the "forty (or even fifty)-somethings" may remember one of the Beatles most memorably playful hits, "When I'm Sixty-Four." To a generation that did not trust *anyone over 30* and certainly could not imagine ever being over 60, the song's subtext—i.e., the notion that *we* might someday be old—was as preposterous as the song was popular. Our culture's obsessions with youth has been frequently decried as one of its saddest and most destructive aberrations. Moreover, in recent years, it has taken an interesting turn as social attitudes equate age with mental incompetence. This circumstance is made all the more difficult when the presumption of incompetence is couched in terms of concern. Good intentions, as we all know, pave the road to hell!

Consider the following situation, which has been related to me by someone whom I trust who swears that it is not exaggerated in any way.

Marie Brown (the name has been changed to protect the well-meaning) is 92 years old. She has lived by herself since her husband died when she was 48. She and her husband had one adopted son who was only 8 when Marie was widowed, so, in an era when most mothers stayed home to rear their children, Marie—unprepared educationally and unsupported socially—had to find a job in a "man's world" to provide for herself and her son. Now, 44 years later, she is fiercely independent and her son struggles to balance his concern for her safety and his own peace of mind.

Over the years, Marie's health has been reasonably good, although she is now suffering from congestive heart failure and arthritis in her knees, which is severe enough to limit her mobility considerably. For this reason, she uses a walker—and moves very, very slowly. To ease her son's worried mind, Marie consented to participating in the "Life-line" program, so, in addition to his own frequent calls and visits, someone calls her daily to check on her safety.

One evening not long ago, Marie, dressed only in her nightgown and slippers, decided to "cook-up" a snack for herself before she went to bed. The grease in the frying pan overheated and caught on fire. Marie went to work immediately: she found the baking soda in the cupboard and dumped it in the frying pan, smothering the fire. She then carefully removed the pan from the stove and placed the pan carefully in the sink.

> **The notion that we might someday be old was as preposterous as the song was popular.**

The real crisis

All of this, of course, took a considerable amount of time because Marie moves very, very slowly. The crisis averted, this should have been the end of it—certainly for a younger person, it would have been—however, a number of coincidences converged to complicate things significantly:

1. At about the time the fire started, "Lifeline" called. Marie, completely—and appropriately—focused on putting out the fire, did not answer the phone.

2. "Lifeline" called its backup person who began calling Marie continuously.

3. "Lifeline" also notified Marie's son and her case manager.

4. The son called a close relative who lived nearby who promised to get over to Marie's home immediately. He also called the police.

5. The smoke alarm in Marie's apartment (Marie lives in a four-apartment building) alerted neighbors, who called the fire department and—concerned that Marie get out in time, started pounding on her door.

...An equal and opposite reaction

Now, consider Marie's predicament. She is trying to put out a small fire, lest it become a bigger one. Her phone is ringing incessantly, the smoke alarm is blaring, people are yelling and banging on her door and police and fire department sirens are screeching louder and louder as they approach her home.

Despite all this, Marie remained focused, and as soon as the fire was contained, she took stock of the situation. Remember, Marie moves very, very slowly. Moreover, she was out of breath from so much activity. However, when she heard the firemen talking about taking an axe to her door, she tried to rush and ended up tipping her walker and falling. Although she was not injured, getting up off the floor is a long and laborious project for her.

Fortunately, Marie's son arrived before the door was "axed," whipped out his key and opened the door in a somewhat more sedate fashion. Hoards of people swept into Marie's small apartment, scooped her off the floor and placed her on the couch. She was flustered and overwhelmed by the sheer presence of so many people—relatives, friends, neighbors, police officers and firemen in full regalia (axes still in hand). Not only was she embarrassed by all the fuss, but she was sitting in front of heaven-only-knows-how-many-people in her nightgown.

Her son, seeing how agitated she was, assumed that she was "confused." To check this assumption, he knelt at her side and said, "Mom, do you know who I am?" Insulted by the implication that she did not know him, she threw him a LOOK and said, "Of course I do!" He countered with, "Well then, who am I?" Marie had had enough. In her most sarcastic tone she said, "Santa Claus," and refused to speak again.

Being elderly does not equate with being incompetent, and begin unable to move quickly does not necessarily equate with being "unsafe" in one's own home.

The crowd of professionals and concerned others continued to question her, and insisted that she get up and walk. Everyone seemed to have an opinion about how to proceed, and each raised his respective voice in an attempt to have his opinion heard above the others. Everyone talked about her, above her and around her as if she did not exist. This made Marie very angry indeed, and even more obstinate. In light of her stony silence and lack of response, the collective wisdom of the crowd was to whisk Marie away to the nearest hospital while arrangements were made to place her in a residential facility.

...to the rescue

At this critical juncture, Marie's professional nurse case manager arrived, chased the entire crowd out onto the front lawn, and in the relative silence that followed, she sat down next to Marie who said, "I am NOT an idiot." The case manager said, "I know that, but I will not be able to overrule that crowd out there unless you help me." "They have no business barging in here, bossing me around." The case manager said, "You are right, Marie, they don't have any right to do this. But they do have the power. And they have good intentions that they intend to demonstrate by taking you to the hospital if you cannot get up and demonstrate that you can walk."

At that, Marie demanded her walker, refused to let the case manager help her get up, and—every inch the grande dame—demonstrated that she was unhurt and could walk, however slowly. "Just how could all those 'men' think that I would get up and parade around in front of them in my nightgown?" she said, very tartly indeed. A brief examination confirmed Marie's demonstration: she was unhurt.

When the case manager went outside to report this happy news, all were relieved, but her well-intentioned benefactors still argued that Marie should be "put" somewhere to keep her safe. Only after considerable discussion wherein the case manager—by now it was almost 9 p.m.—explained that even younger people can have kitchen fires (she, herself, dealt with several, and more than a few burnt meals, as a newlywed not so many years ago!) did the neighbors disburse, the police return to their vehicles and the firemen roll up their hoses and secure their axes. Then, and only then, was the case manager able to sit down with Marie's son and discuss more moderate approaches to her care and safety.

Of safety and rights

Being elderly does not equate with being incompetent, and begin unable to move quickly does not necessarily equate with being "unsafe" in one's own home. Marie had a minor fire, which she handled appropriately. Because of circumstances beyond her control, matters got out of hand. She was embarrassed enough to begin with, but when her own son—not to mention the hoard of strangers—humiliated her by treating her "like an idiot" (her own term), she was angry...and perhaps she had a right to be angry. Age ought not to deprive one of the right to freedom, adult prerogatives and lifestyle choices.

Because she knew Marie, her situation and her son—and because of her credibility with them and with the professional community—Marie's case manager was able to resolve a chaotic situation. Incidentally, she also prevented an injustice and saved Medicare (parts A and B) a not inconsiderable sum of money.

Credible, clinically competent and compassionate nurse case managers pave the road to success—clinically and financially—for today's health and human services networks. Without them, even with the best intentions, we may find ourselves "on the road to hell."

February 1995

INDEX

A

Abortion, 231
Advance directives, 91-93
Advanced licensure, 55-60
Advanced practice nurses, 290
Agency for Health Care Policy and
  Research, 61
Aging, 231, 337-341
AIDS, 45-50, 231
American Association of Critical Care
  Nurses, 6
American Hospital Association, 9
American Medical Association, 9, 10-11,
  20, 45, 148, 248, 250, 290
American Nurses Association, 3, 6, 10-11,
  45, 55, 148, 152, 290
American Organization of Nurse
  Executives, 15
Angelou, Maya, 71-72
Artificial organs, 40
Associate-degree programs, 7-10
Austin, J.A., 95, 103
Ayala, Marissa, 84-87

B

Baccalaureate programs, 7-10
Barton, Clara, 124
Bigotry, 113-118
Blanchfield, Florence A., 23
Block, Gay, 101
Bone marrow transplantation, 84-87
Breckinridge, Ann, 124
Bryant, L. Edward, 13

C

Camus, Albert, 94
Cardiopulmonary resuscitation, 15-16
Cassell, Eric, 90
Centers for Disease Control, 47-49
Certification, 148
Change
  leadership and, 132-133, 211-214
  technology and, 134-135
Clinton, Bill, 19, 20, 151, 247, 248, 256-
  259, 294
Clinton, Hillary, 152
Collegiality, 42-44
Communication
  computers and, 40
  with words, 143-147
Confidentiality, 94-97

Continuous quality improvement, 100,
  122, 314
Corporate Culture, 186-192
Corporations, ethical, 111-112
Creative thinking, 173
Critical care nurses, 36-37
Critical pathways, 14-15, 76
Cross-training, 74
Cruzan, Nancy Beth, 78-83, 91-92

D

de Galard-Terrause, Genevieve, 23, 124
Diagnostic Related Groups (DRGs), 11,
  12-13
Dickens, Charles, 164
Diploma education, 7-10
Dix, Dorothea Lynde, 23
DNA probes, 40
Douglas, Frederick, 117
Drucker, Malka, 101

E-F

Edison, Thomas, 282-284
Education of nurses, 7-10
Emerson, Ralph Waldo, 30
Empowerment, 207-210
Endoscopy, 40
Entry into practice, 7-10
Envy, 119-124
Ethical issues
  bone marrow transplantation, 84-87
  cardiopulmonary resuscitation, 15-16
  confidentiality, 94-97
  dying infants, 16-19
  mercy killing, 53, 125-130, 231
  professionalism and, 105
  right to die, 78-83
  right to privacy, 94-97
  right to refuse treatment, 91-93
  suicide, 128-130, 231
Excellence, origins of, 43-44
Fried, Charles, 96

G

Genetic engineering, 40
Global budgets, 20, 21
Goldsmith, Charles, 144-145